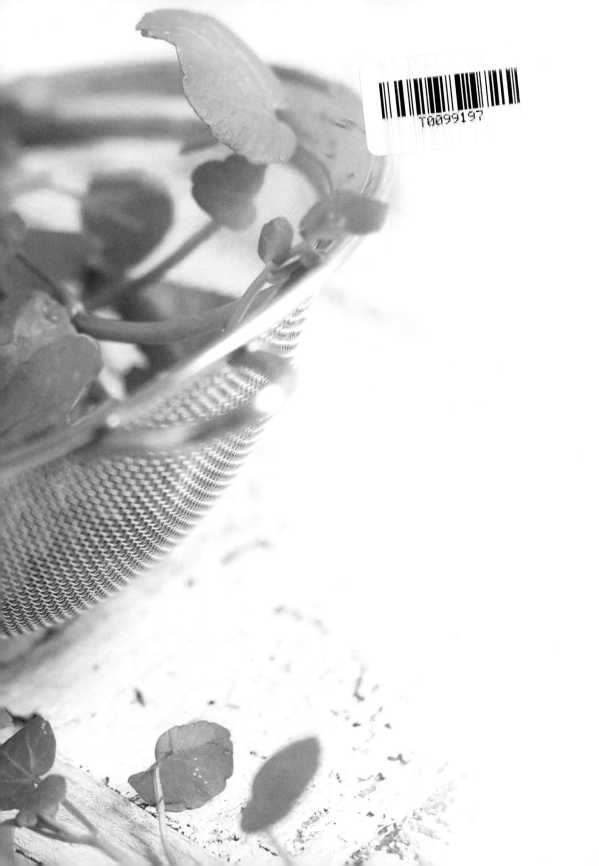

SLIM & FIT
IN 21 DAYS

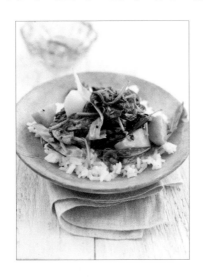

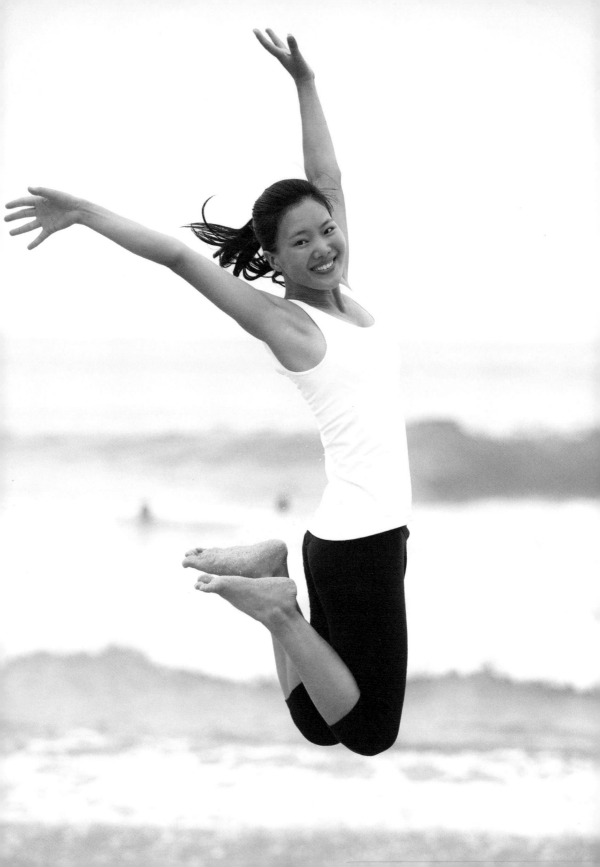

SLIM & FIT IN 21 DAYS

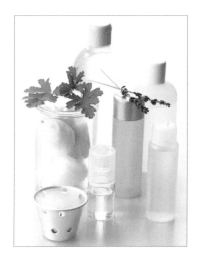

- **Three-week diet and exercise plan**
- **Feel healthier and look fabulous**
- **Delicious easy-to-follow recipes**

LUCY DONCASTER

LORENZ BOOKS

This edition is published by Lorenz Books,
an imprint of Anness Publishing Ltd
info@anness.com
www.lorenzbooks.com, www.annesspublishing.com
twitter: @AnnessBooks

If you like the images in this book and would like to investigate
using them for publishing, promotions or advertising, please visit
our website www.practicalpictures.com for more information.

A CIP catalogue record for this book is available from
the British Library.

Publisher: Joanna Lorenz
Editor and designer: Lucy Doncaster
Contributors: Jane Collins, Sally Norton, Kate Shapland and
  Nicky Pope
Photography: Simon Bottomley, Nick Cole, Michelle Garrett,
  Christine Hanscomb, Alistair Hughes, Liz McAulay and
  David Goldman

Publisher's Note
Although the advice and information in this book are believed to
be accurate and true at the time of going to press, neither the
authors nor the publisher can accept any legal responsibility or
liability for any errors or omissions that may have been made nor
for any inaccuracies nor for any loss, harm or injury that comes
about from following instructions or advice in this book.

CAUTION
It is advisable to consult a qualified medical professional before
undertaking any exercise or dieting regimes – especially if you have
a medical condition or are pregnant.

Cook's Notes
• Bracketed terms are intended for American readers.
• For all recipes, quantities are given in metric and imperial
measures and, where appropriate, in standard cups and
spoons. Follow one set of measures, not a mixture, because
they are not interchangeable.
• Standard spoon and cup measures are level. 1 tsp = 5ml,
1 tbsp = 15ml, 1 cup = 250ml/8fl oz.
• Australian standard tablespoons are 20ml. Australian
readers should use 3 tsp in place of 1 tbsp for measuring
small quantities.
• American pints are 16fl oz/2 cups. American readers should
use 20fl oz/2.5 cups in place of 1 pint when measuring
liquids.
• Electric oven temperatures in this book are for conventional
ovens. When using a fan oven, the temperature will need to
be reduced by 10–20°C/20–40°F. Since ovens vary, you
should check with your manufacturer's instruction book for
guidance.
• The nutritional analysis given for each recipe is calculated
per portion (i.e. serving or item), unless otherwise stated. The
analysis does not include optional ingredients, such as salt
added to taste.
• Medium (US large) eggs are used unless otherwise stated.

CONTENTS

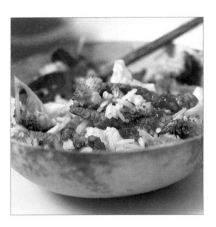

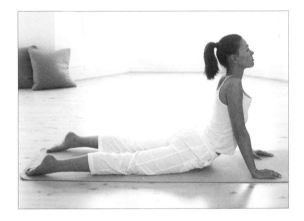

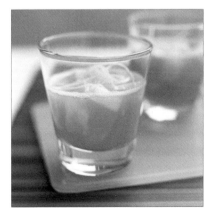

INTRODUCING THE NEW YOU

We all know that being fit is one of the best ways to improve our long-term health, but sometimes it is hard to get motivated. This book aims to help you lose weight, improve your fitness and make the most of your natural assets, all in just 21 days. There are no food exclusions, no hunger – just easy-to-follow diet and exercise regimes and beauty advice that will give visible results, quickly.

Losing a little weight is something that many of us aspire to, and achieving this is actually fairly simple, on paper at least: your body needs to burn off more calories than it consumes. This means that both the quantity and the quality of the foods eaten need to be monitored, and in this book a suggested daily allowance of 1,200Kcal is given, with recipes containing minimal saturated fat. If you wish to lose more weight, you can take a more radical approach, for instance consume just 500Kcal on two non-consecutive days in a week. Make sure you do not do rigorous aerobic exercise on these days or you could faint; stretching and toning exercises are best.

Alongside this calorie-controlled diet plan is an exercise programme that aims to burn off calories, as well as tone specific areas that often need a little work. If you follow the plan, the results will be visible within just three weeks, and since you will be eating a range of healthy foods, you will notice the benefits on the inside as well as the outside.

EAT YOURSELF SLIM

When trying to reduce your calorie intake what you eat is just as important as how much. A balanced, healthy diet that leaves you satisfied and energized is much better than a deprivation regime, which is harder to maintain and often fails to provide all the nutrients you need.

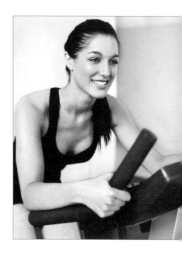

Above A healthy diet, regular exercise and simple beauty routines will leave you looking and feeling glowing and energized.

With this in mind, the meal planners have been carefully put together to include a wide range of delicious dishes that are packed with flavour but low in calories. The recipe section contains more than 80 mouthwatering dishes, many of which are quick and easy to create and you can mix and match to devise your own menus, if you like.

In addition to at-a-glance calorie and saturated fat counts next to the recipe names, full nutritional information is also given and, where carbohydrates such as pasta or noodles can be swapped for zero-calorie versions, the calorie count for this variation is provided. This is useful if you plan to restrict your intake to 500Kcal on two days in a week as it will enable you to adapt the planners and recipes to suit your requirements.

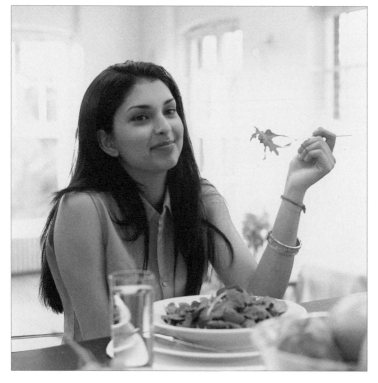

Left Losing weight should be an enjoyable experience, involving delicious as well as nutritious meals at regular intervals.

CAUTIONS

• If you are pregnant, are on any medication or suffer from any illness, consult your doctor before you begin any diet.

• Take things easy and build up your exercise routines gradually, particularly if you haven't done any exercise for quite a while.

• It is normal for your heart to beat faster and for you to become breathless during sustained aerobic exercise. Stop immediately if you feel nauseous, dizzy, light-headed, experience severe breathlessness, chest pain, pain in your neck and arms, or heart palpitations.

• If after taking regular exercise and making other lifestyle changes you still feel chronically tired, consult a doctor.

ENERGIZING EXERCISE

Exercise that gets your heart beating faster and develops your lung capacity – aerobic exercise – gives you energy and zest for life, helps you to reduce and then maintain a healthy body weight, and can be fun!

If you usually feel fatigued and never seem to get enough sleep, the last thing you probably feel like doing is exercising. Indeed, you may feel that an exercise routine will use up what little bit of spare energy you have – but really the complete opposite is true. Regular aerobic exercise will give you lots more energy and reduce the need for sleep. You are likely to sleep better, wake up feeling fresher and have more stamina to cope with everything the day throws at you.

HOW MUCH EXERCISE?

For visible results in just three weeks you should make sure you do 30 minutes' aerobic exercise – which uses the most calories and helps burn off fat – for five days in every week. Use the remaining two days to stretch and tone and perhaps treat yourself to some beauty treatments. The planners give specific times for aerobic exercises, while the other activities all take about 10 minutes each to complete.

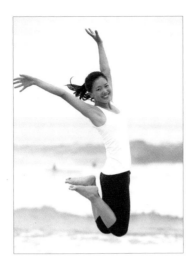

Above Being fit and healthy will give you a renewed zest for life and set you on the road to a brighter, more invigorated future.

If you are new to exercise, take things fairly slowly at first and build up your stamina, endurance and energy levels gradually. If you are very unfit it would be a good idea to improve your fitness slightly before you start the diet by going power-walking or swimming a few times a week, so you are physically and mentally prepared for the more strenuous activity outlined in the programmes and will be more likely to stick to the regime.

Once the three-week period is over, try to maintain the habit of exercising regularly – 30 minutes' exercise three to four times a week is generally recommended in order to maintain fitness levels and a healthy weight.

LOOK AS GOOD AS YOU FEEL

The last sections of the book are devoted to bodycare and haircare. Packed with top tips, step-by-step techniques and recipes for home-made beauty treatments, these chapters will help you to make the most of your natural assets. From pampering your skin, dealing with problem areas and giving your nails a once-over to buying and applying make-up and caring for your hair, these chapters will arm you with all the skills you need to complete the transformation into a new you!

10 REASONS FOR LOSING WEIGHT AND EXERCISING

• **You will look better** – Exercise will make you look firmer, slimmer and better, both in and out of your clothes. Exercise improves posture, too.

• **You will be happier** – Doing vigorous exercise for at least 10 minutes on a regular basis will help to trigger the production of endorphins, which are your body's feel-good chemicals.

• **You will burn up calories** – Exercising will help you lose weight and keep you at your ideal weight. Just 30 minutes, or three 10-minute blocks, of continuous exercise will get your heart pumping faster. This will increase your metabolic rate and help you burn fat faster, even when you've stopped exercising.

• **You will suffer less from stress** – Exercise can help to reduce stress, tension and stress-related problems such as headaches and insomnia.

• **You will have more resistance to illnesses** – Aerobic exercise reduces the risk of heart disease, bowel disease, diabetes, strokes and osteoporosis. Exercise boosts the immune system and helps you to fight off colds and flu.

• **You will have more energy** – You will notice an improvement in your energy levels in as little as one week if you take regular exercise. After three weeks you should have improved your strength.

• **You will have great skin** – Exercise makes your skin glow because it improves your circulation. It improves the appearance of cellulite, too.

• **You will feel more confident** – Looking better, feeling stronger, having more energy and being more able to deal with stress – all these benefits of exercise will make you feel confident.

• **You will feel more alert** – Exercise makes you mentally fitter. It increases the supply of oxygen and glucose to the brain, which improves concentration.

• **You will be helping family and friends** – Increasing your fitness can improve the health of your family and friends. Encourage them to work out with you or make exercise a social event.

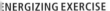

FOLLOWING A WEIGHT-LOSS REGIME

When following a 21-day programme, you will need to incorporate the plans into your daily routine so that the changes to your diet and lifestyle are relatively easy to make and adhere to. Plan for all eventualities, where possible, so your weight-loss regime runs as smoothly as possible and think about the three-week period as just the start of a whole new way of living.

It is worth letting family members know that you are planning to undertake a diet and fitness regime and set aside enough time to cook healthy recipes and fit in the exercises. It is best to keep your diary relatively clear in the evenings, when you may want to exercise and have control over what you eat. Late nights and alcohol will also do your motivation the next day no good at all.

Once you have completed the 21-day plan, try not to slip back into old habits; continue to eat healthily and exercise regularly in order to maintain the benefits gained by following the healthy living guidelines.

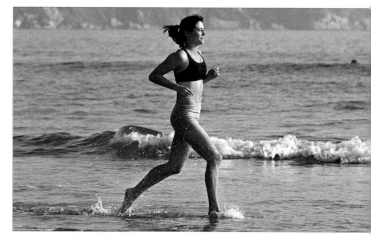

FLEXIBLE EATING
Menu plans are suggested in this book, although you can vary the recipes, swap meals around and substitute ingredients to suit your own preferences and according to availability. However, be sure to choose a variety of dishes to ensure that you get a balance of food groups, and be aware that changing ingredients will affect the calorie and fat counts, which can make gauging your daily intake harder. To make the suggested plans easier to follow, most of the recipes use commonly found ingredients and frozen fruit and vegetables can often be substituted when fresh foods are not available.

Above Fit in exercise at a time and in a location that suits you. First thing in the morning may be best for some people.

PLAN MEAL AND EXERCISE TIMES
Eat three meals a day – breakfast, lunch and dinner. Do not skip any meals and make time for breakfast. Even if you do not feel hungry in the morning and do not usually eat breakfast, get into the habit of doing so. There are lots of delicious choices suggested in the chapter on 'Juices, smoothies and breakfast ideas'. Breakfast kick-starts the metabolism after resting overnight and the body needs fuel for energy so that you do not feel tired and unable to concentrate.

Eating regularly also helps to keep your blood sugar levels stable and can prevent binge eating or snacking between meals. Aim to have breakfast before 9am, lunch between midday and 2pm and dinner before 8pm, allowing a reasonable time between meals for

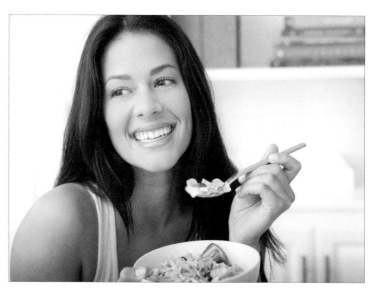

Left Do not be tempted to skip breakfast – it is vital for stabilizing blood sugar levels and will prevent you snacking mid-morning.

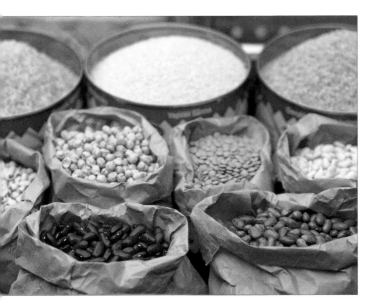

Left Stock up on an assortment of healthy ingredients such as lentils, beans, peas and wholegrains before you start the diet plan.

A NEW START FOR ALL THE FAMILY

The recipes in this book can be useful for helping all of the family to follow a healthier diet. They encourage the use of a wide range of different fruits and vegetables, wholegrains and fish, in preference to highly processed and refined foods, which are usually loaded with unhealthy fats, sugar, salt and chemical additives as well as being low in fibre. Bear in mind, however, that a weight-loss diet is not suitable for children as they need more fat than adults and they should eat the correct amount of calories for their age. If a famiy member is ill, pregnant or has special dietary requirements then you should stick to the guidelines given by a health professional for them.

To avoid cooking different meals for every family member, remove your portion first, then add bread, pasta, meat and dairy products to their portions afterwards if necessary, although most dishes are suitable for everyone. Or, make a batch just for yourself, split it into portions and freeze or refrigerate it for another time. If you follow a diet with a partner or friend then so much the better, as you will spur each other on and can share the cooking.

DIETING TIPS

• It is best to avoid dieting during times of high stress, such as when moving house, starting a new job or when a relationship breaks down. You need to be able to devote quite a bit of time to cooking and exercising and external distractions make the process much harder, especially if they mean you cannot control your daily schedule.

• Set yourself an achievable target – you can lose weight and tone up in 21 days but you won't drop four dress sizes!

comfortable digestion. If you have a busy schedule, try to arrange appointments around mealtimes rather than letting your diary rule when you have time to eat.

Have a clear idea of which exercises you are going to do each day and try to ensure you leave enough time to do them. If for some reason you cannot do the planned aerobic exercise – if a meeting overruns and it is too dark to go for a walk or run by the time you get home, for nstance – then be flexible and look at the alternative aerobic routines outlined n this book. So long as you do 30 minutes of aerobic exercise five days in each week and cut your calorie intake, you will continue to lose weight.

BE PREPARED

Keep the kitchen cupboards well stocked with staples such as rice, beans, lentils, canned tomatoes, nuts and dried fruit, so that you always have the basics to hand for making a healthy meal. Also keep a selection of frozen fruit and vegetables, fresh home-made stock, fish and chicken in the freezer. Read through the recipes and buy ingredients that keep well so that you are prepared if you don't have much time to shop, and make some dishes ahead and store them in the refrigerator or freezer for days when you are short of time.

Make sure you have all the sports equipment you are going to require before you start the 21-day regime, and invest in a good pair of trainers if you plan to do impact sports such as running. It is also a good idea to read through the section on beauty and stock up on any creams, lotions, essential oils and bathtime aids such as loofahs that you think you will need. Allow some me-time on the days when you are not doing any exercise and indulge in a facial, hair masque or manicure after a long soak in the bath. You will have earned it!

Right Wearing appropriate clothing and well-fitting trainers designed for sport is very important when doing exercise.

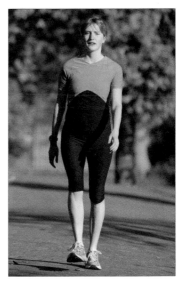

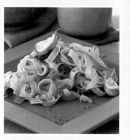

	MONDAY 1,246 Kcal	**TUESDAY** 1,266 Kcal	**WEDNESDAY** 1,238 Kcal

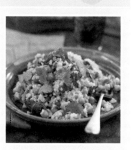 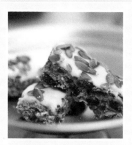 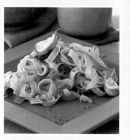

BREAKFAST & SNACKS

MONDAY
- Traditional Scottish Porridge (p30) – 115Kcal
- 1 banana – 105Kcal
- white tea or coffee – 15–20Kcal

TUESDAY
- 2 slices toast with butter and jam – 250Kcal
- white tea or coffee – 15–20Kcal
- Date Slice (p67) – 198Kcal

WEDNESDAY
- Popped Amaranth Cereal (p30) – 28Kcal
- 115g/4oz/½ cup yogurt – 65Kcal
- 1 banana – 105Kcal
- white tea or coffee – 15–20Kcal

LUNCH & SNACKS

MONDAY
- Winter Farmhouse Soup (p36) – 266Kcal
- Flaxseed Quinoa Muffin (p66) – 287Kcal

TUESDAY
- Artichoke and Cumin Dip (p32) – 76Kcal
- 5 breadsticks – 100Kcal
- Courgette and Bean Salad (p42) – 183Kcal

WEDNESDAY
- Spicy Red Lentil Soup (p35) – 203Kcal
- 1 wholemeal (whole-wheat) pitta bread – 181Kcal
- Orange Oatie (p66) – 110Kcal

EVENING MEAL

MONDAY
- Bulgur Wheat with Lamb (p62) – 366Kcal
- Tropical-scented Fruit Salad (p64) – 87Kcal

TUESDAY
- Cod, Tomato and Pepper Stew (p57) – 312Kcal
- 115g/4oz blueberries – 62Kcal
- 115g/4oz/½ cup low-fat yogurt – 65Kcal

WEDNESDAY
- Tagliatelle with Veg Ribbons (p48) – 348Kcal
- 50g/2oz green salad – 8Kcal
- 25g/1oz/¼ cup unsalted mixed nuts – 170Kcal

EXERCISES

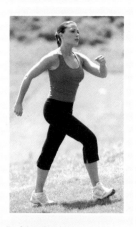 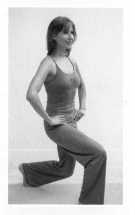 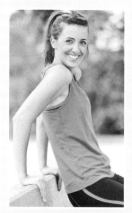

MONDAY
Total time: 80 minutes
- Start-up Moves (p76)
- Power-walking for 30 minutes (p80)
- Trimmer Arms (p94)
- Waist Workshop (p100)
- Spine Thrillers (p107)
- Stretch Slimmer (p103)

TUESDAY
Total time: 70 minutes
- Start-up Moves (p76)
- Machine Workout for 30 minutes (p83) OR a running programme (pp81–2) if you do not have access to a machine
- Better Buttocks (p95)
- Inner Thigh Tone (p96)
- Super Shoulders (p93)

WEDNESDAY
Total time: 80 minutes
- Total-body Warm-up (88)
- Upper Body Tone (p91)
- Lower Body Tone (p92)
- Leaner Legs (p98)
- Ballet Style (p102)
- Back Basics (p106)
- Cooling Down (p86)
- Facial Workout (p109)

THURSDAY 1,245 Kcal	**FRIDAY** 1,185 Kcal	**SATURDAY** 1,235 Kcal	**SUNDAY** 1,310 Kcal

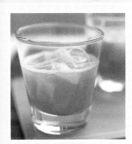 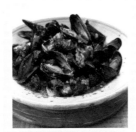 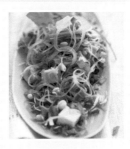 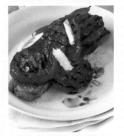

THURSDAY

- 30g/generous 1oz/1⅓ cups bran flakes with milk – 157 Kcal
- 25g/1oz/⅛ cup raisins – 85Kcal
- 1 banana – 105Kcal
- white tea or coffee – 15–20Kcal

- Bulgur Wheat Salad (p40) – 149Kcal
- Chewy Fruit Slice (p31) – 110Kcal
- Pineapple and Ginger Juice (p28) – 120Kcal

- Five-spice Beef in Bean Sauce (p63) – 399Kcal
- 50g/2oz broccoli – 18Kcal
- 50g/2oz carrots – 17Kcal
- 115g/4oz/½ cup yogurt – 65Kcal

FRIDAY

- Apple and Quinoa Breakfast Bar (p31) – 174Kcal
- Wheatgrass Tonic (p28) – 36Kcal

- Mussels in Tomato Broth (p38) – 211Kcal
- 1 wholemeal (whole-wheat) pitta bread – 146Kcal
- 1 apple – 51Kcal

- Spiced Vegetables Over Rice (p44) – 345Kcal
- Poached Pumpkin (p65) – 157Kcal
- 115g/4oz/½ cup yogurt – 65Kcal

SATURDAY

- Apricot and Ginger Smoothie (p29) – 167Kcal
- 115g/4oz/½ cup yogurt – 65Kcal
- 115g/4oz/⅔ cup berries – 32Kcal
- white tea or coffee – 15–20Kcal

- Noodle, Tofu and Bean Salad (p43) – 132Kcal
- 25g/1oz/⅛ cup ready-to-eat dried apricots – 47Kcal
- 25g/1oz/⅛ cup seeds – 150Kcal

- Chicken on Pitta (p59) – 408Kcal
- Warm Aubergine Salad (p41) – 102Kcal
- Carob and Cherry Cookie (p67) – 112Kcal

SUNDAY

- Lime and Watermelon Tonic (p28) – 114Kcal
- Griddled Tomatoes on Toast (p30) – 172Kcal
- white tea or coffee – 15–20Kcal

- Mushroom Soup (p34) – 58Kcal
- 2 wholemeal (whole-wheat) pitta breads – 292Kcal
- Aubergine Dip (p33) – 129Kcal
- 1 banana – 105Kcal

- Chinese Fish and Tofu Stew (p55) – 238Kcal
- 50g/2oz/¼ cup brown rice – 182Kcal

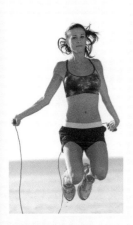 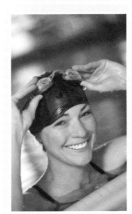 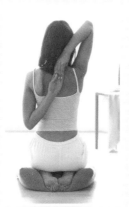 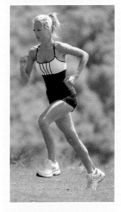

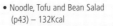

THURSDAY

Total time: 70 minutes
- Start-up Stretches (p77)
- Burn Fat Faster (p78)
- Dance Moves (p79)
- Skipping Fit (p81)
- Outer Thigh Tone (p97)
- Toned Stomach (p101)
- Cooling Down (p86)

FRIDAY

Total time: 50 minutes
- Water Workout (p85), to include 20 minutes swimming laps as well as the 10 minutes of aqua exercises
- Spine Thrillers (p107)
- Stretch It Out (p105)

SATURDAY

Total time: 50 minutes
- Total-body Warm-up (p88)
- Effortless Exercise (p89)
- Ballet Style (p102)
- Back Basics (p106)
- Facial Workout (p109)

SUNDAY

Total time: 80 minutes
- Start-up Moves (p76)
- Running for 30 minutes (pp81–2)
- Trimmer Arms (p94)
- Super Shoulders (p93)
- Chest Exercises (p99)
- Cooling Down (p86)

MEAL & EXERCISE PLANNERS – WEEK 2

	MONDAY 1,157 Kcal	**TUESDAY** 1,231 Kcal	**WEDNESDAY** 1,156 Kcal
	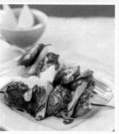	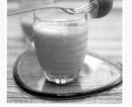	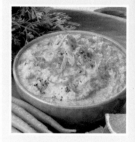
BREAKFAST & SNACKS	• 45g/2oz muesli (granola) with semi-skimmed milk – 216Kcal • 250ml/8fl oz/1 cup fresh orange juice – 108Kcal • white tea or coffee – 15–20Kcal	• 2 slices toast with butter and jam – 250Kcal • Mango and Lime Lassi (p29) – 71Kcal • 25g/1oz/⅕ cup seeds – 150Kcal	• Traditional Scottish Porridge (p30) – 115Kcal • 1 banana – 105Kcal • 250ml/8fl oz/1 cup fresh orange juice – 108Kcal
LUNCH & SNACKS	• Sushi-style Tuna Cubes (p38) – 153Kcal • Grilled Skewered Chicken (p39) – 165Kcal • 1 flatbread – 90Kcal	• Vegetables in Ginger Broth (p35) – 77Kcal • 1 apple – 51Kcal • Carob and Cherry Cookie (p67) – 112Kcal	• Baked Chickpea Samosas (p37) – 119Kcal • Spiced Carrot Dip (p33) – 60Kcal • 1 flatbread – 90Kcal • 1 orange – 62Kcal
EVENING MEAL	• Ratatouille (p47) – 140Kcal • baked potato – 156Kcal • 30g/1oz/¼ cup half-fat mature (sharp) Cheddar cheese – 77Kcal • 115g/4oz/⅔ cup berries – 32Kcal	• Thai Scallops with Chilli Quinoa (p52) – 422Kcal • 150g/6oz greens (collards) – 36Kcal • 115g/4oz/1 cup blueberries – 62Kcal	• Beef and Mushroom Burger (p63) – 211Kcal • 150g/6oz new potatoes – 105Kcal • Apricot and Ginger Compote (p65) – 181Kcal
EXERCISES	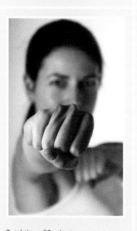	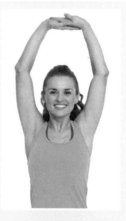	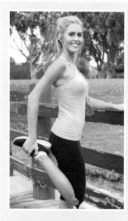
	Total time: 60 minutes • Start-up Moves (p76) • Skipping Fit (p81) • Putting Up a Fight (p84) • Burn Fat Faster (p78) • Lower Body Tone (p92) • Cooling Down (p86)	Total time: 50 minutes • Water Workout (p85), to include 20 minutes swimming laps as well as the 10 minutes of aqua exercises • Spine Thrillers (p107) • Stretch It Out (p105)	Total time: 60 minutes • Total-body Warm-up (p88) • Minimal Moves (p104) • Trimmer Arms (p94) • Spine Thrillers (p107) • Essential Relaxation (p108) • Facial Workout (p109)

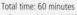

THURSDAY 1,182 Kcal	**FRIDAY** 1,165 Kcal	**SATURDAY** 1,207 Kcal	**SUNDAY** 1,268 Kcal

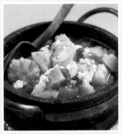 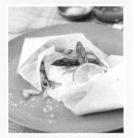 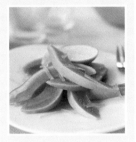 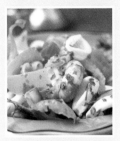

- 30g/generous 1oz/1⅓ cups bran flakes with milk – 157 Kcal
- 25g/1oz/⅙ cup raisins – 68Kcal
- 1 banana – 105Kcal
- white tea or coffee – 15–20Kcal

- Popped Amaranth Cereal (p30) – 28Kcal
- 115g/4oz/½ cup yogurt – 65Kcal
- Pineapple and Ginger Juice (p28) – 120Kcal

- Griddled Tomatoes on Toast (p30) – 172Kcal
- Lime and Watermelon Tonic (p28) – 114Kcal
- white tea or coffee – 15–20Kcal

- 2 slices toast with butter and jam – 250Kcal
- white tea or coffee – 15–20Kcal

- Miso Broth with Tofu (p34) – 71Kcal
- 2 slices wholemeal (whole-wheat) bread – 170Kcal
- Apricot and Ginger Smoothie (p29) – 167Kcal

- Beetroot and Yogurt Salad (p41) – 95Kcal
- 2 flatbreads – 180Kcal
- Flaxseed Quinoa Muffin (p66) – 287Kcal

- Thai Fish Soup (p36) – 65Kcal
- 75g/3oz/¾ cup grapes – 60Kcal
- 1 banana – 105Kcal
- Chewy Fruit Slice (p31) – 110Kcal

- Warm Seafood and Herb Salad (p42) – 184Kcal
- 1 wholemeal (whole-wheat) pitta bread – 181Kcal
- 1 banana – 105Kcal

- Squash, Potato and Corn Stew (p50) – 329Kcal
- green leafy salad – 8Kcal
- Tropical-scented Fruit Salad (p64) – 87Kcal

- Steamed Red Snapper (p54) – 110Kcal
- 150g/6oz new potatoes – 105Kcal
- 50g/2oz broccoli – 18Kcal
- Poached Pumpkin (p65) – 157Kcal

- Indian Chicken Stew (p60) – 308Kcal
- 50g/2oz/¼ cup white rice – 198Kcal
- Papaya, Lime and Ginger Salad (p64) – 55Kcal

- Penne with Vegetable Sauce (p49) – 401Kcal
- 115g/4oz/1 cup blueberries – 62Kcal
- 115g/4oz/½ cup yogurt – 65Kcal

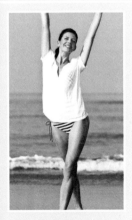 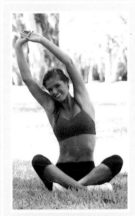 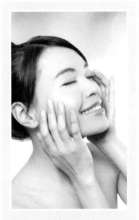 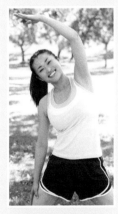

Total time: 70 minutes
- Start-up Moves (p76)
- Machine Workout for 30 minutes (p83) OR a running programme (pp81–2) if you do not have access to a machine
- Better Buttocks (p95)
- Leaner Legs (p98)
- Cooling Down (p86)

Total time: 80 minutes
- Start-up Stretches (p77)
- Power-walking for 30 minutes (p80)
- Trimmer Arms (p94)
- Toned Stomach (p101)
- Spine Thrillers (p107)
- Stretch Slimmer (p103)

Total time: 40 minutes
- Work Workout (p90)
- Stretch It Out (p105)
- Essential Relaxation (p108)
- Facial Workout (p109)

Total time: 80 minutes
- Start-up Moves (p76)
- Running for 30 minutes (pp81–2)
- Better Buttocks (p95)
- Outer Thigh Tone (p97)
- Waist Workshop (p100)
- Cooling Down (p86)

MEAL & EXERCISE PLANNERS – WEEK

MONDAY 1,219 Kcal	TUESDAY 1,112 Kcal	WEDNESDAY 1,255 Kcal

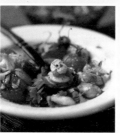 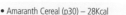 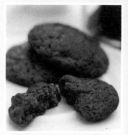

BREAKFAST & SNACKS

• 50g/2oz/½ cup muesli (granola) with semi-skimmed milk – 216Kcal • Pineapple and Ginger Juice (p28) – 120Kcal • coffee or tea – 15–20Kcal	• Amaranth Cereal (p30) – 28Kcal • 115g/4oz/½ cup yogurt – 65Kcal • 1 banana – 105Kcal • Lime and Watermelon Tonic (p28) – 114Kcal	• 2 slices toast with butter and jam – 250Kcal • 250ml/8fl oz/1 cup fresh orange juice – 108Kcal • coffee or tea – 15–20Kcal

LUNCH & SNACKS

• Seared Thai Beef Salad (p43) – 174Kcal • Flaxseed Quinoa Muffin (p66) – 287Kcal • 1 apple – 51Kcal	• Vegetables in Ginger Broth (p35) – 77Kcal • 2 slices wholemeal (whole-wheat) bread – 170Kcal • Date Slice (p67) – 198Kcal	• Spring Vegetable Omelette (p51) – 187Kcal • Roasted Peppers (p40) – 134Kcal • Mango and Lime Lassi (p29) – 71Kcal

EVENING MEAL

• Butter bean and Tomato Stew (p45) – 138Kcal • 1 wholemeal (whole-wheat) pitta bread – 181Kcal • 115g/4oz/1 cup berries – 32Kcal	• Fried Rice with Beef (p62) – 232Kcal • 150g/5oz greens (collards) – 36Kcal • Tropical-scented Fruit Salad (p64) – 87Kcal	• Spanish-style Vegetables (p44) – 185Kcal • 75g/3oz/¾ cup pasta – 188Kcal • Carob and Cherry Cookie (p67) – 112Kcal

EXERCISES

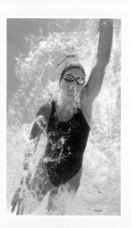 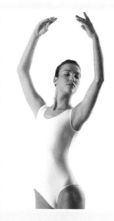 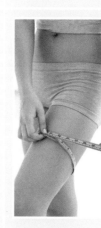

Total time: 50 minutes • Water Workout (p85), to include 20 minutes swimming laps as well as the 10 minutes of aqua exercises • Spine Thrillers (p107) • Facial Workout (p109)	Total time: 70 minutes • Total-body Warm-up (88) • Upper Body Tone (p91) • Lower Body Tone (p92) • Leaner Legs (p98) • Ballet Style (p102) • Stretch Slimmer (p103) • Cooling Down (p86)	Total time: 80 minutes • Start-up Moves (p76) • Running for 30 minutes (pp81–2) • Better Buttocks (p95) • Outer Thigh Tone (p97) • Waist Workshop (p100) • Cooling Down (p86)

| **THURSDAY** 1,243 Kcal | **FRIDAY** 1,353 Kcal | **SATURDAY** 1,255 Kcal | **SUNDAY** 1,181 Kcal |

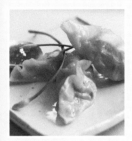 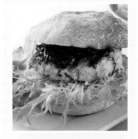 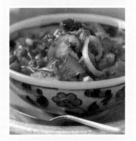 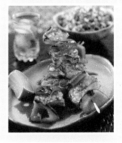

- 30g/generous 1oz/1⅓ cups bran flakes with milk – 157 Kcal
- Pineapple and Ginger Juice (p28) – 120Kcal

- Steamed Crab Dim Sum (p39) – 166Kcal
- Mushrooms with Chilli Sauce (p37) – 40Kcal
- 25g/1oz/¼ cup nuts – 170Kcal

- Tamarind Fish Stew (p56) – 317Kcal
- 50g/2oz/¼ cup brown rice – 182Kcal
- 150g/5oz greens (collards) – 36Kcal
- Papaya, Lime and Ginger Salad (p64) – 55Kcal

- Apricot and Ginger Smoothie (p29) – 167Kcal
- 115g/4oz/½ cup yogurt – 65Kcal
- 115g/4oz/1 cup berries – 32Kcal
- coffee or tea – 15–20Kcal

- Spring Vegetable Stir-fry (p49) – 358Kcal
- Flaxseed Quinoa Muffin (p66) – 287Kcal
- 1 orange – 62Kcal

- Turkey Patties (p58) – 146Kcal
- 50g/2oz broccoli – 18Kcal
- 50g/2oz carrots – 17Kcal
- Apricot and Ginger Compote (p65) – 181Kcal

- Griddled Tomatoes on Toast (p30) – 172Kcal
- 250ml/8fl oz/1 cup fresh orange juice – 108Kcal
- coffee or tea – 15–20Kcal

- Ceviche (p54) – 145Kcal
- 1 flatbread – 90Kcal
- 75g/3oz/¾ cup grapes – 60Kcal
- Apple and Quinoa Breakfast Bar (p31) – 174Kcal

- Lentils with Mushrooms (p46) – 242Kcal
- 50g/2oz/¼ cup brown rice – 182Kcal
- 115g/4oz/1 cup blueberries – 62Kcal

- Traditional Scottish Porridge (p30) – 115Kcal
- 1 banana – 105Kcal
- Wheatgrass Tonic (p28) – 36Kcal

- Beetroot and Yogurt Salad (p41) – 95Kcal
- Aubergine Dip (p33) – 129Kcal
- 2 flatbreads – 180Kcal
- Chewy Fruit Slice (p31) – 110Kcal

- Prawn and Pepper Kebabs (p53) – 102Kcal
- Spicy Squid (p53) – 122Kcal
- Tofu and Pepper Kebabs (p51) –187Kcal

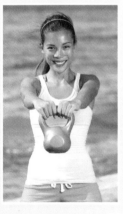 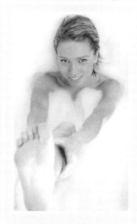 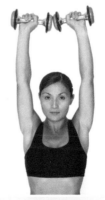 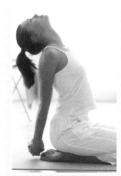

Total time: 60 minutes
- Start-up Moves (p76)
- Skipping Fit (p81)
- Putting Up a Fight (p84)
- Burn Fat Faster (p78)
- Upper Body Tone (p91)
- Stretch It Out (p105)

Total time: 60 minutes
- Effortless Exercise (p89)
- Leaner Legs (p98)
- Stretch Slimmer (p103)
- Spine Thrillers (p107)
- Essential Relaxation (p108)
- Facial Workout (p109)

Total time: 70 minutes
- Start-up Moves (p76)
- Machine Workout for 30 minutes (p83) OR a running programme (pp81–2) if you do not have access to a machine
- Trimmer Arms (p94)
- Super Shoulders (p93)
- Cooling Down (p86)

Total time: 80 minutes
- Burn Fat Faster (p78)
- Dance Moves (p79)
- Skipping Fit (p81)
- Better Buttocks (p95)
- Outer Thigh Tone (p97)
- Toned Stomach (p101)
- Chest Exercises (p99)
- Cooling Down (p86)

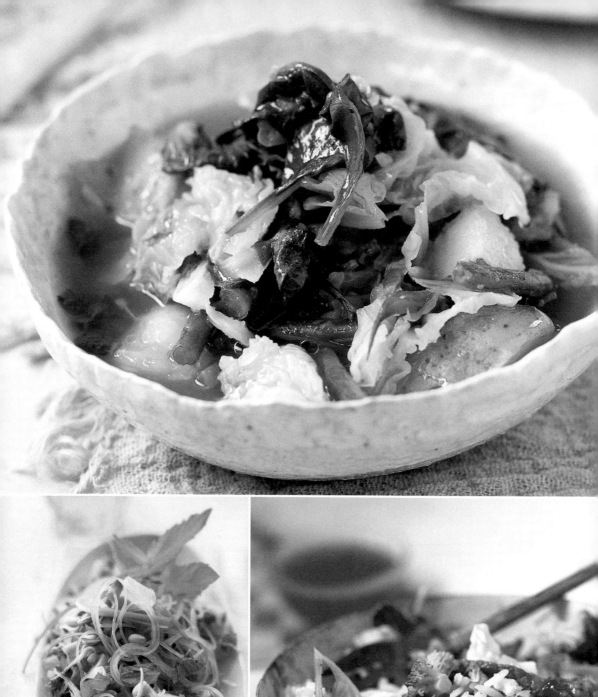
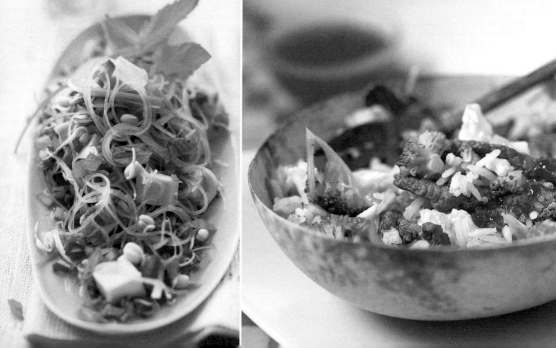

HEALTHY WEIGHT LOSS IN 21 DAYS

Developing healthy eating habits plays a huge part in how your body performs and how you feel about it. Choosing foods that promote good health makes sense, and is surprisingly simple. So take control of your food intake to improve your diet, your health and your beauty.

A HEALTHY BALANCE

When trying to lose weight it is important that your body receives the correct nutrition and that you don't exclude foods that help you to function properly. These pages give an overview of the most important vitamins, minerals and food groups and how these can be incorporated into a healthy diet

Balance is crucial to healthy eating, and understanding how to choose a healthy combination of foods is the first step towards improving your eating habits and lifestyle.

VITAL VITAMINS
Vitamins are crucial for a number of processes carried out by the body. Usually only a few milligrams are required each day but they are essential for good health. Most vitamins cannot be made by the body so they must be obtained from food.

Vitamins have a wide variety of functions in the body. Some play a part in enzyme activity. Enzymes are protein molecules and they are responsible for every aspect of metabolism, the energy we produce. Producing plenty of enzymes

improves the processes of digestion, detoxification and immunity, and also helps to slow down the aging process. Vitamins A, C and E are antioxidants that protect body cells from damage. If the body is under stress, vitamin C (ascorbic acid) is used more quickly. Smoking is a form of stress for the body, and smokers should be particularly careful to make sure that they eat fruit and vegetables containing vitamin C.

ESSENTIAL MINERALS
A wide variety of minerals is vital for good health, growth and body functioning. Some, such as calcium and iron, are needed in quite large amounts, and for some people there is a real risk of deficiency if they do not eat a healthy diet that is high in these minerals.

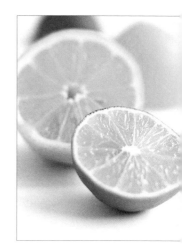

Above Citrus fruits are a rich source of vitamin C. One orange a day provides an adult's daily requirement of the vitamin.

VITAMINS	BEST SOURCES	ROLE IN HEALTH
A (retinol – animal foods, beta-carotene – plant foods)	Milk, butter, cheese, egg yolks, margarine, carrots, apricots, squash, red (bell) peppers, broccoli, green leafy vegetables, mango and sweet potatoes.	Essential for vision, bone growth, and skin and tissue repair. Beta-carotene acts as an antioxidant and protects the immune system.
B1 (thiamin)	Wholegrain cereals, brewer's yeast, potatoes, nuts, beans, peas and lentils, and milk.	Essential for energy production, the nervous system, muscles and heart. Promotes growth and boosts mental ability.
B2 (riboflavin)	Cheese, eggs, milk, yogurt, fortified breakfast cereals, yeast extract, almonds and pumpkin seeds.	Essential for energy production and for the functioning of vitamin B6 and niacin as well as tissue repair.
Niacin (part of B complex)	Pulses (legumes), potatoes, fortified breakfast cereals, wheatgerm, peanuts, milk, cheese, eggs, peas, mushrooms, green leafy vegetables, figs and prunes.	Essential for healthy digestive system, skin and circulation. It is also needed for the release of energy.
B6 (piridoxine)	Eggs, wholemeal (whole-wheat) bread, breakfast cereals, nuts, bananas, and cruciferous vegetables such as broccoli.	Essential for assimilating protein and fat, to make red blood cells, and for a healthy immune system.
B12 (cyanocobalamin)	Milk, eggs, fortified breakfast cereals, cheese and yeast extract.	Essential for formation of red blood cells, maintaining a healthy nervous system and increasing energy levels.
Folate (folic acid)	Green leafy vegetables, fortified breakfast cereals, bread, nuts, beans, peas and lentils, bananas and yeast extract.	Essential for cell division. Extra is needed pre-conception and during pregnancy to protect against neural tube defects.
C (ascorbic acid)	Citrus fruits, melons, strawberries, tomatoes, broccoli, potatoes, peppers and green vegetables.	Essential for the absorption of iron, and for healthy skin, teeth and bones. An antioxidant that strengthens bones.
D (calciferol)	Sunlight, margarine, vegetable oils, eggs, cereals and butter.	Essential for bone and teeth formation. Helps the body to absorb calcium and phosphorus.
E (tocopherol)	Seeds, nuts, vegetable oils, eggs, wholemeal bread, green leafy vegetables, oats and cereals.	Essential for healthy skin, circulation and maintaining cells – an antioxidant.

ight Not all fats are 'bad' for you, but only mall amounts are needed to stay healthy. at monounsaturated fats such s olive oil, and polyunsaturates such as unflower oil rather than saturated fats.

alcium: A regular supply of calcium is ital because bone tissue is constantly eing broken down and rebuilt. A alcium-rich diet is particularly important uring adolescence, pregnancy, reastfeeding, the menopause and old ge. Smoking, lack of exercise, too much lcohol, high protein and high salt ntakes all encourage calcium losses.

on: Only a fraction of the iron present in ood is absorbed, although it is much more eadily absorbed from red meat than from egetable sources. Vitamin C also helps vith absorption. Pregnant women, women vho have heavy periods and vegetarians specially require an adequate intake.

race elements: These include other ssential minerals such as zinc, iodine, nagnesium and potassium. Although mportant, they are needed in only minute uantities. They are found in a variety of oods and deficiency is very rare.

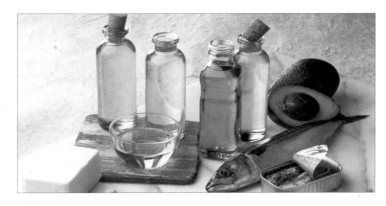

FATS – GOOD AND BAD

Eggs, butter, milk and meat are a good source of energy, but we tend to eat too much fat, which is why many of us are overweight. Cut down on fat in your diet but do not cut it out completely: eat less red meat and more fish and poultry; grill (broil), bake or stir-fry (using polyunsaturated and monounsaturated oils); eat eggs in moderation; and use semi-skimmed (low-fat) or skimmed milk. Use margarine, or switch to a reduced-fat olive-oil spread instead of butter; reserve it for special occasions.

Saturated fats come mainly from animal products (milk, butter, cheese and meat) and in excess are thought to contribute to raised cholesterol levels. The recipes in this book all contain less than 5g saturated fat.

Polyunsaturated fats are found in vegetable oils such as sunflower, safflower, corn and soya-bean oils, as well as some fish oils and nuts, and are said to help lower cholesterol levels.

Mono-unsaturated fats are found in olive and rapeseed oils; they are also said to lower cholesterol levels.

MINERALS	BEST SOURCES	ROLE IN HEALTH
Calcium	Milk, cheese, yogurt, green leafy vegetables, sesame seeds, broccoli, dried figs, pulses, almonds, spinach and watercress.	Essential for building and maintaining bones and teeth, muscle function and the nervous system.
Iron	Red meat, egg yolks, fortified breakfast cereals, tofu, leafy vegetables, dried apricots, pulses, wholegrains.	Essential for healthy blood and muscles.
Zinc	Peanuts, wholegrains sunflower and pumpkin seeds, beans, peas and lentils, milk, hard cheese and yogurt.	Essential for a healthy immune system, tissue formation, normal growth, wound healing and reproduction.
Sodium	Most of the salt we eat comes from processed foods such as crisps (US potato chips), cheese and canned foods. It is also found naturally in most foods.	Essential for nerve and muscle function and the regulation of body fluid.
Potassium	Bananas, milk, beans, peas and lentils, nuts, seeds, wholegrains, potatoes, fruits and vegetables.	Essential for water balance, normal blood pressure and nerve transmission.
Magnesium	Nuts, seeds, wholegrains, pulses, tofu, dried figs and apricots, and vegetables.	Essential for healthy muscles, bones and teeth, normal growth and nerves.
Phosphorous	Milk, cheese, yogurt, eggs, nuts, seeds, beans, peas and lentils, and wholegrains.	Essential for healthy bones and teeth, energy production and the assimilation of nutrients.
Selenium	Avocados, lentils, milk, cheese, butter, brazil nuts and seaweed.	Essential for protecting against free radical damage and may protect against cancer.
Iodine	Seaweed and iodized salt.	Aids the production of hormones released by the thyroid gland.
Chloride	Table salt and foods that contain salt.	Regulates and maintains the balance of fluids in the body.
Manganese	Nuts, wholegrains, beans, peas and lentils, tofu and tea.	Essential component of various enzymes that are involved in energy production.

CEREAL GRAINS

The seeds of cereal grasses, grains are packed with concentrated goodness and are an important source of complex carbohydrates, protein, vitamins and minerals. As an added bonus, grains are inexpensive and versatile.

Eat plenty of wholegrain foods such as brown rice, wholemeal (whole-wheat) bread, wholemeal flour and wholemeal pasta; they are a much better choice than refined types.

FRUIT AND VEGETABLES

Make a habit of eating lots of fresh fruit and vegetables: these are rich in carbohydrates, vitamins and minerals. Nutritionists recommend that every day you should aim to eat seven to ten portions of fruit (one portion could be a medium apple or orange, a wine glass of fruit juice, two plums or kiwi fruit or one large slice of melon or pineapple) and vegetables (aim to eat two large spoonfuls of vegetables – fresh, frozen, or tinned – with your main meal).

Fruit and vegetables contain phytochemicals, the plant compounds that stimulate the body's enzyme defences against carcinogens (the

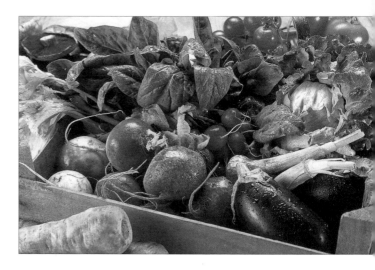

substances that cause cancer). The best sources are broccoli, cabbages, kohlrabi, radishes, cauliflower, brussels sprouts, watercress, turnips, kale, pak choi (bok choy), mustard greens, spring greens (collards), chard and swede (rutabaga).

PULSES, SEEDS AND NUTS

As well as being economical, pulses (legumes) are easy to cook and good to eat. Low in fat and high in complex carbohydrates, vitamins and minerals,

Above One of the easiest ways to boost your intake of fibre, vitamins and minerals is to eat plenty of vegetables.

they are a valuable source of protein and good for diabetics, as they help to control sugar levels. You can buy dried ones, then soak and cook them at home or, for convenience, use canned ones. Check the label of cans and get ones that are stored in water, without the addition of salt or sugar.

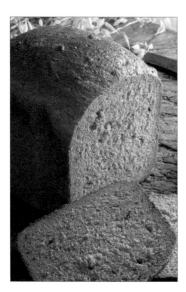

Above Starchy carbohydrates are high in fibre and low in fat and provide energy for exercise while on the diet.

FACTS ON FIBRE

Fibre is important for a healthy diet. Your body cannot digest it, so, in rather basic terms, it goes in and comes out, taking other waste with it. Fibrous foods include bread, rice, cereals, vegetables, fruit and nuts. Aim for about 30g (just over 1oz) of fibre a day. These are some examples of good sources:

GOOD SOURCES	AVERAGE PORTION	GRAMS OF FIBRE
Wholemeal (whole-wheat) pasta	75g/3oz/¾ cup (uncooked)	9
Baked beans	115g/4oz/scant 1 cup	8
Frozen peas	75g/3oz/¾ cup	8
Bran flakes	50g/2oz/2 cups	7
Blackberries	90g/3½oz/scant 1 cup	6
Raspberries	90g/3½oz/scant 1 cup	6
Muesli (granola)	50g/2oz/½ cups	4–5
Baked potato (with skin)	150g/5oz	3.5
Banana	average fruit	3.5
Brown rice	50g/2oz/¼ cup	3
Cabbage	90g/3½oz	3
Red kidney beans	40g/1½oz/¼ cup	3
Wholemeal bread	1 large slice	3
High-fibre white bread	1 large slice	2
Stewed prunes	6 fruit	2

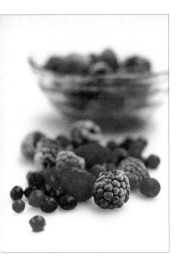

Seeds and nuts are a good source of B vitamins and vitamin E, an antioxidant that has been associated with a lower risk of heart disease, stroke and certain cancers. They are also a useful source of protein, especially for vegetarians, but are high in calories and fat.

SUGARY FOODS
Many of us tend to eat too much sugar to try drastically reducing the amount of added sugar in your diet for 21 days (your body will still obtain it naturally from certain vegetables and fruit) and see how you feel. Craving sugary foods when you are pre-menstrual is common, to eat little and often; snack on fruit with a high water content, such as watermelon and strawberries. If you really need a pick-me-up, choose one of the recipes for healthier low-fat bakes.

SALTY ISSUES
It is generally a good idea to eat less salt as too much may lead to high blood pressure. There are some low-sodium salts available, so use these if you choose to season food with salt. Do not buy salted butter, avoid processed and smoked cheeses, add just a little salt (or none at all) to cooking water, and avoid processed foods.

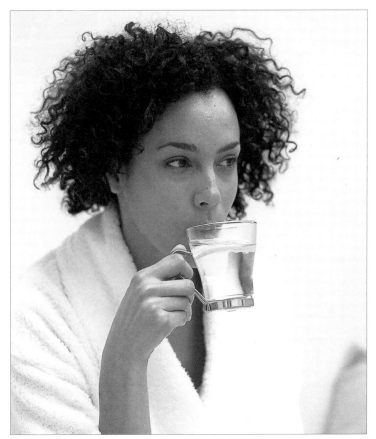

Above As a rough guide you should aim to drink at least eight glasses of fluid every day to keep your body properly hydrated.

FLUID INTAKE
Drink plenty of liquid: your body loses 2–3 litres/3–5 pints of water every day, so drink no less than 1.5 litres/2½ pints of fluid daily. Herbal and regular tea, coffee and other liquids all count, but it is best to avoid alcohol during the 21-day programme since this contains empty calories and will make exercising the next day harder.

You will need to drink plenty of extra water straight after exercise in order to rehydrate and, if you can, try to sip from a water bottle while you are out running, power-walking or cycling. Drinking caffeine, such as black coffee, about an hour before exercise can improve your performance and help you to keep going for longer.

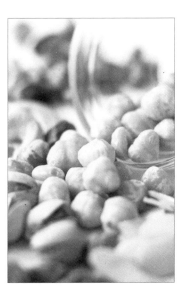

Above Nuts and seeds are nutritious and delicious and provide a range of vitamins, but be aware that they are calorific.

HEALTHY SHOPPING

Supermarkets offer a fabulous range of foods, but faced with such an array it is easy to be distracted by offers on unhealthy or convenience foods, and to forget about seasonality and the provenance of the items. Fortunately, just a little thought will enable you to make better, healthier choices.

It is easy to become fixated on food when you are dieting, but this is not always helpful as obsessing about eating can make you more hungry! Roaming around a supermarket on an empty stomach is also not advised, as you can easily be lured into snacking, so it may be worth using the Internet to do the majority of your shopping and then topping up on fresh produce at a market, where the produce is likely to be fresher and there are fewer unhealthy temptations. If you do go to a supermarket, write a list before you go and stick to it – this will make the trip quicker and probably cheaper as you whizz round the store collecting only the required ingredients for your planned meals.

SEASONALITY

Although most fresh ingredients are now available all year round, they are at their best nutritionally, and taste infinitely superior, when they are eaten in season. Choosing locally grown foods can be advantageous as they will have lower food miles, but it is not always possible to grow some common, healthy foods, such as citrus or tropical fruits, in every climate. Seasonality is more imporant.

Below Try to buy fruits and vegetables when they are in season and at their best. If they are locally grown, so much the better.

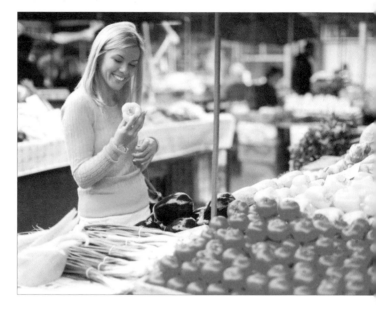

Above Fresh food markets are inspiring places to pick up fresh produce and are often cheaper than supermarkets, too.

BE LABEL-SAVVY

There is much debate about organic and free-range foods, and they can be prohibitively expensive if budgets are tight. They do have their benefits however, so if you adopt an 'eat less, eat better' attitude and have just a small amount of a better-quality item it is often worth paying a little more.

In brief, organic agriculture is a method of farming that avoids the use of pesticides and fertilizers for growing crops, and the routine use of drugs and antibiotics for rearing animals. Strict laws and regulations ensure that these conditions are complied with, and organic producers must be certified by a recognized organization.

Organic farming is more labour intensive so the produce often costs more. However, it does not contain many of the

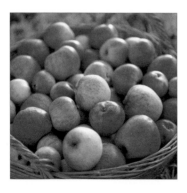

chemical residues found in intensively farmed produce, it tends to be higher in vitamins and minerals, and it also contains higher levels of micro-nutrients believed to offer protection from diseases such as cancer. It may also taste better.

Free-range foods are usually products such as eggs, poultry and meat. In theory, animals should have access to outside space and lead a more natural life than intensively reared animals, although some may spend some time indoors.

Below Fresh, juicy pears make a healthy snack or dessert.

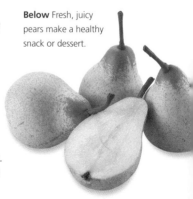

nimals are likely to be treated with
ntibiotics, but they do have a higher
tandard of living and the product may
aste better too.

   Shopping for fish can be difficult as we
re bombarded with often confusing
nformation. In general, wild, line-caught
r hand-dived seafood is a more
esponsible choice than farmed or
rawled produce. Some fish stocks are at
ritical levels, so check websites to see
vhich types are the most sustainable.

   Most countries have various other
chemes and food labels, some of which
nay be a bit misleading, so you should
heck what food labels mean before
naking an informed choice about what
o buy. Remember, too, that while it
nakes sense to choose organic or free-
ange when possible, just eating plenty of
ruit and vegetables is the most
mportant thing for a healthy diet.

Right Include a range of different vegetables
n your diet, whether you are trying to lose
veight or not. In addition to being packed
vith vitamins and minerals, they are high in
ibre and low in calories.

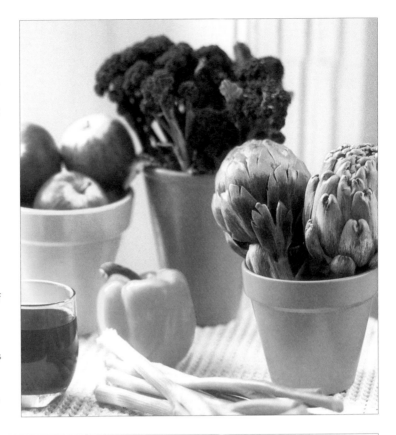

SHOPPING TIPS

• Choose to shop where you know the
food is of a good quality. Independent
shops generally sell fresh produce
supplied by local growers and
producers, and some large
supermarkets are committed to
ensuring their meat, dairy and eggs
comes from producers with high
standards of animal welfare.

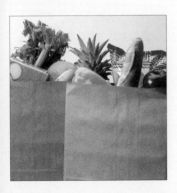

• Shop selectively and plan what you
need. Look at the menus and recipes for
the week and make a note of what
ingredients you will need to buy.
• Take a list and do not shop when you
are hungry, so that you're less likely
to be tempted to buy foods that should
be avoided while following the weight-
loss programme. In some instances you
can be flexible and buy what looks fresh
and appealing. So for example, you
could just list 'fruit for fruit salad', then
decide what to buy when you see what
looks fresh and is in season.
• Try to avoid buying ready-prepared
fruit, vegetables and salads. Not only
will you pay a premium price, but
because they are already cut up, they
will have lost some vitamin value.
• Buy fresh herbs freely, unless of course
you are able to use home-grown ones.
• Buy fresh foods regularly rather than
storing them for long periods.

• Stock up on staples, such as rice,
beans, wholegrains, dried fruits, nuts,
seeds and good quality canned foods
so that you always have ingredients
ready to hand for making a satisfying
and nutritious meal. Wholefood stores
or co-operatives are a good place to buy
a wide variety of dry goods that are of
good quality and reasonably priced.
• Store dry goods in airtight containers
to keep them in peak condition and use
them before their 'best before' date.
• Don't buy anything that is high in
sugar, saturated fat, salt or additives.
Always read labels carefully if you are
unsure, checking the 'per 100g' figures.
• Don't be taken in by terms like
'natural', 'country' or 'traditional' as
they mean little on processed foods.
• Take durable shopping bags with you;
reuse paper and plastic bags or buy
mesh bags that zip shut that you can
use again and again.

EATING FOR WEIGHT LOSS

People tackle weight loss in ways that suit their lifestyles. But the safest and best way to shift excess pounds in the long as well as the short term is to combine regular exercise with a balanced calorie-controlled diet that contains all the components your body requires.

What you eat when you are trying to lose weight should not be that different from a normal eating plan – except for the amount you consume. If you have only a small amount to lose and you cut your calorie intake from the recommended 2,000Kcal per day, to 1,200Kcal per day, you will lose weight. If you are aiming to lose a significant amount, you can take a more radical approach, which involves consuming no more than 500Kcal on two non-consecutive days in a week.

Your basic weight-loss ethos, whatever the daily calorie consumption, is less sugar and saturated fats and more fibre and starch; the calories you eat should come from foods that supply you with the right number of nutrients to keep your body functioning properly.

MIND OVER MATTER

Quick weight loss is inspiring, but it is important to think ahead too; you need to retain your palate and eating habits and reassess your physical activity so that you

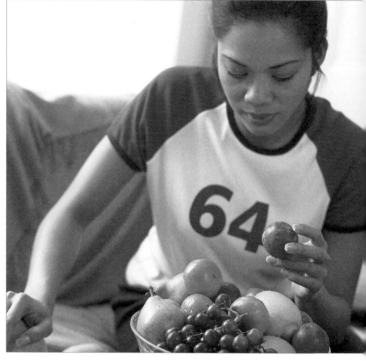

can lose weight and stay slim. You cannot expect to achieve miracles in a few days, but you will see a difference within three weeks if you eat properly and exercise regularly. Losing weight successfully is like getting fitter: you need a horizon – or goal – ahead of you to help spur you on.

HEALTHY WEIGHT LOSS

To lose weight you have to eat fewer calories than your body burns up every day, but this varies from person to person. The exact amount depends on your personal composition – how much fat your body has, your metabolism and how much you weigh to begin with. As a rule of thumb though, the heavier you are when you start slimming, the more weight you are likely to lose within 21 days or a month. When you lose weight it comes off all areas of your body, but it can

Above Fruit is the ideal snack when you are dieting. It is very low in fat and calories and provides vitamins and minerals.

take longer to shift from certain areas, such as your arms and legs. This is where exercise is particularly helpful, because working on trouble spots will encourage the weight to come off more quickly.

HEALTHY EATING HABITS

If you start the day with a substantial breakfast your body will get all the energy it needs early on. It is also true that those who fail to eat something sustaining for breakfast are more likely to snack mid-morning and this is often not a good nutritional choice. A bowl of muesli (granola) or porridge with fruit is a good slow-release option.

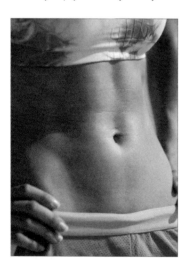

Above Regular aerobic and toning exercise is the best way to achieve your dream figure.

ight Fruit and vegetable juices are packed with goodness, flush out the digestive system and encourage the elimination of toxins. Be ware that they may be high in calories.

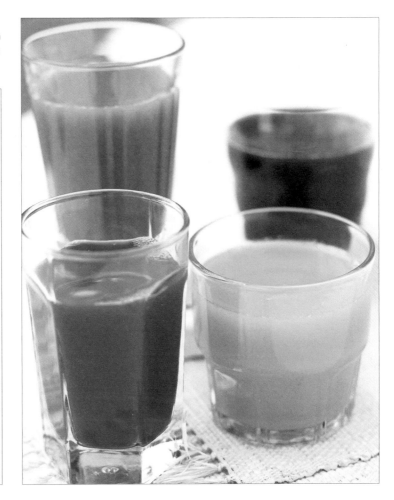

TIPS FOR WEIGHT LOSS

• If you can, it is better to eat before 8pm to give you energy and time to burn off the calories.

• Do not be tempted to skip meals as this will make you crave and overeat at the next meal, and it slows down your metabolism, which ultimately hinders weight loss.

• Eat little and often to stop hunger pangs and keep blood sugar steady.

• Drink lots of water.

• If you want to snack, keep a supply of fruit, raw vegetables and raisins nearby.

• Don't be tempted to take slimming pills, diuretics or laxatives to speed up weight loss; they upset the body's natural equilibrium – something that can take a long time to rebalance.

• Exercise regularly; activity uses up calories, and this is key to weight loss.

• Don't give up if you lapse: it is quite normal to veer off track every so often, and as long as you get back on course as soon as you can, all your hard work will not be ruined.

You are most likely to succeed in changing your diet in the long term if you eat regularly, in moderation, and slowly – and savour every mouthful. Although the bonuses of eating in a balanced way do not come instantly, if you take stock now and concentrate on eating wholesome fresh foods, as well as avoiding high-fat, sugar-rich foods such as cakes, pastries and salty snacks, you will probably notice a marked difference in your energy levels within a couple of weeks.

If your energy levels take a dive because your blood sugar is low, don't reach for chocolate or a rich biscuit (cookie). The quick energy boost these give will be followed by a slump, and you may end up far more tired than you were at the start. Eat a wholemeal

(whole-wheat) salad sandwich instead; the carbohydrate in the bread will give you a more efficient energy fix that will be more prolonged and even.

WEIGHT GAIN AND GIVING UP SMOKING

You may put on a small amount of weight at first, but if you are a smoker then making the decision to stop is the biggest leap you can make towards living a healthier lifestyle. If you think that kicking the smoking habit will make you pick at food all day, keep raw vegetables and very low-calorie foods such as rice cakes to hand to munch on. Speak to a health professional for further advice – they are there to help you give up and a fear of weight gain is simply not an excuse not to do it.

GAUGING WEIGHT LOSS

You may choose to weigh yourself once a week. First thing in the morning is best. Drawing up a goal chart to record any weight losses (and gains) may help to keep you inspired. Don't weigh yourself too often because you are more likely to get discouraged; once a week is enough. Or, if you prefer, ignore the scales and focus on how you feel by keeping a check on how your clothes fit. When tight clothes become more comfortable this is a sign that you are losing weight. Alternatively, keep a record of your measurements (bust, waist and hips) and see how they alter over the 21-day period. Do whatever works best for you, and when you have lost a little weight reward yourself with a treat such as a manicure or massage.

KNOW YOUR CALORIE COUNTS

When calorie counting it is important to account for everything you eat, including accompaniments and healthy snacks, as well as drinks. Here is a list of the calorie counts for some common foods, but you should also check the packet as counts can vary from brand to brand and according to size:

FOOD TYPE	PORTION/QUANTITY	KCAL
Long-grain white rice (uncooked)	50g/2oz/¼ cup	198Kcal
Long-grain brown rice (uncooked)	50g/2oz/¼ cup	182Kcal
Boiled new potatoes	150g/6oz	105Kcal
Boiled old potatoes	150g/6oz	136Kcal
Baked potato	115g/4oz	156Kcal
White pasta (raw weight)	50g/2oz/½ cup	188Kcal
Wholemeal (whole-wheat) pasta (uncooked)	50g/2oz/½ cup	158Kcal
Zero-calorie pasta	50g/2oz/½ cup	2Kcal
Cooked egg noodles	50g/2oz/½ cup	215Kcal
Zero-calorie noodles	50g/2oz/½ cup	2Kcal
Medium-sliced white bread	1 slice/36g/1½oz	78Kcal
Medium-sliced wholemeal bread	1 slice/36g/1½oz	85Kcal
Toast with butter and jam	1 slice/36g/1½oz	125Kcal
Flatbread	x1/85g/3oz	90Kcal
White pitta bread	x1/85g/3oz	124Kcal
Wholemeal pitta bread	x1/85g/3oz	146Kcal
Plain breadstick	1	20Kcal
Plain thin rice cake	1	19Kcal
Carrot sticks	50g/2oz	18Kcal
(Bell) pepper strips	50g/2oz	14Kcal
Celery sticks	50g/2oz	5Kcal
Cooked broccoli	50g/2oz	18Kcal
Cooked carrots	50g/2oz	17Kcal
Cooked greens (collards)	50g/2oz	14Kcal
Green leafy salad	50g/2oz	8Kcal
Low-fat natural (plain) yogurt	115g/4oz/½ cup	65Kcal
Banana	1 medium fruit	105Kcal
Apple	1 medium fruit	51Kcal
Orange	1 medium fruit	62Kcal
Strawberries, raw, fresh	115g/4oz/⅔ cup	32Kcal
Blueberries, raw, fresh	115g/4oz/1 cup	62Kcal
Raisins	25g/1oz/⅕ cup	68Kcal
Dried apricots	25g/1oz/⅛ cup	47Kcal
Mixed nuts, unsalted	25g/1oz/¼ cup	170Kcal
Mixed seeds	25g/1oz/⅕ cup	150Kcal
Muesli (granola) with semi-skimmed milk	50g/2oz/½ cup	216Kcal
Bran flakes with semi-skimmed milk	30g/generous 1oz/1⅓ cups	157Kcal
Fresh orange juice	250ml/8fl oz/1 cup	108Kcal
Black coffee	250ml/8fl oz/1 cup	10Kcal
White coffee with semi-skimmed milk	250ml/8fl oz/1 cup	20Kcal
Latte, regular	250ml/8fl oz/1 cup	136Kcal
Cappuccino, whole milk	250ml/8fl oz/1 cup	125Kcal
Tea with semi-skimmed milk	250ml/8fl oz/1 cup	15Kcal
Red wine	120ml/4fl oz/½ cup	85Kcal
White wine	120ml/4fl oz/½ cup	90Kcal
Lager	300ml/10fl oz/1¼ cups	160Kcal

EATING OUT

The best way to solve the problem of dining out without lapsing – and without drawing attention to yourself and still being able to enjoy yourself – is as follows:
• Order a salad appetizer.
• Skip bread or breadsticks.
• Drink just one glass of wine, along with lots of water.
• Choose a simple main course, such as grilled (broiled) fish or chicken; avoid rich sauces and dishes containing butter.
• Skip dessert and instead finish with herbal tea or choose espresso or black coffee, not cappuccino.

MAXIMIZING NUTRITIONAL VALUE

To obtain the most nutritional value from your food, especially fruit and vegetables, it should be as fresh as possible, and its preparation or cooking should ensure that as many nutrients as possible are retained.
• Make sure your supplier has a rapid turnover. Check foods before you buy.
• Transport produce home quickly. Remove any plastic wrapping. Store in a cool larder or in the refrigerator crisper.
• Avoid buying fresh produce from a store that has fluorescent lighting over displays, as this can cause a chemical reaction that depletes the nutrient levels in fruit and vegetables.
• Avoid peeling fruit and vegetables if you can, since nutrients are concentrated just below the skin.

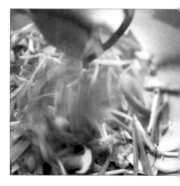

Above Heat the wok or frying pan over a high heat before adding the vegetables, and keep the food moving all the time.

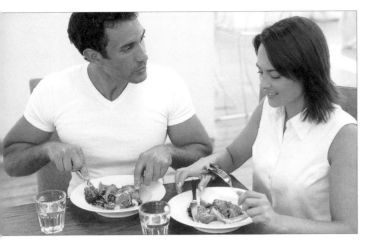

When eating out while dieting, opt for grilled (broiled) fish or chicken and plenty of salad, and choose water over wine.

STEAMING

This method of cooking is nutritionally excellent as the food does not come in to direct contact with the water, so few soluble nutrients are lost and the flavour and texture of the food is retained. Also, no oil or fat is needed. There are many types of steamer available, including electrical tiered steamers, insert pans with a stepped base that will fit on top of any pan, or Chinese-style bamboo or expanding steamer baskets, which are placed above a pan of simmering water, or you can improvise with a foil-covered wire strainer. Steaming is also the ideal way to prepare most fish, as the delicate flesh requires only the gentlest cooking.

stead wash it thoroughly and don't
eel or slice produce until you are
eady to use it.

Try to eat the majority of your
egetables and fruit raw. Otherwise,
se a steamer in preference to boiling.

Buy nuts and seeds in small
uantities and store them in airtight
ontainers in a cool, dark place. Herbs,
pices, pulses (legumes), flours and
rains should be kept in the same way.

TIR-FRYING

n excellent method for preserving
aximum nutrients, stir-frying is a
reat way to rustle up a healthy, low-
at meal in a very short space of time –
deal after a workout in the evening.

Peel and chop all the ingredients
to bitesize pieces before you start
ooking so that they are ready for use
nd they cook quickly and evenly. Place
hem in piles so that you can add them
o the wok or frying pan in the order of
heir cooking time – crunchy vegetables
uch as carrots and baby corn first,
hen quick-cooking vegetables such as
ell) peppers and mangetouts (snow
eas), and finally leafy vegetables.

The best technique is to place the
vok or frying pan over the heat
vithout any oil. When the pan is hot,
ribble drops of oil, necklace fashion,
n to the inner surface just below the
im. As the drips slither down into the
an, they coat the sides, then puddle in
he base. You can get away with using

just about a teaspoon of oil if you
follow this method. Add the food to be
cooked when the oil is very hot, and
keep it moving using two spatulas or
spoons, as when tossing a salad.

VEGETABLE STOCK

Home-made stock is often used to add extra flavour to soups and stews. However, bought stock (bouillon) cubes, and powder and chilled stocks from the supermarket are often high in salt and may contain flavour enhancers and other artificial additives. The best option, therefore, especially whether on a diet or just trying to eat well, is to make your own stock so you can be sure of what goes into it. It is easy to make using a selection of vegetables, with fresh herbs added for flavour and black pepper for seasoning.

Makes 1 litre/1¾ pints/4¼ cups
750g/1lb 10oz vegetables (such as
  onions, leeks, celery, carrots,
  fennel, swede (rutabaga), turnip,
  squash, broccoli and mushrooms),
  trimmed, peeled if necessary,
  and chopped
a bunch of fresh herbs (such as bay
  leaf, thyme, oregano, rosemary,
  tarragon or parsley stalks)
a large strip of lemon rind
6 black peppercorns

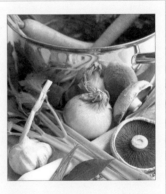

1 Put all the ingredients in a large pan and pour over 1.5 litres/2½ pints/ 6¼ cups of cold water. Bring to the boil, then reduce the heat, partially cover and simmer for about 40 minutes.

2 Remove from the heat, strain the stock through a sieve (strainer) or colander and discard the vegetables.

3 Leave to cool, then pour into a plastic container. Keep chilled in the refrigerator and use within 4 days, or store in the freezer for up to 6 months. Thaw in a microwave or slowly in a pan, before using.

JUICES, SMOOTHIES & BREAKFAST IDEAS

LIME AND WATERMELON TONIC
114KCAL, 0.3G SAT FAT

This refreshing juice will help to cool the body, calm the digestion and cleanse the system. The real magic, however, lies in its flavour. The light watermelon taste is fresh on the palate, while the honey warms the throat, and the tart lime gives it an edge.

1 watermelon
1 litre/1¾ pints/4 cups chilled water
juice of 2 limes
clear honey, to taste
ice cubes, to serve
Serves 4

1 Using a sharp knife, chop the watermelon into chunks, cutting off the skin and discarding the black seeds.

2 Place the watermelon chunks in a large bowl, pour the chilled water over and leave to stand for 10 minutes.

3 Strain the watermelon chunks, then push them through a juicer or blend in a blender.

4 Stir in the lime juice and sweeten to taste with honey. Pour into a jug (pitcher), add ice cubes and stir. Serve in wide, chunky glasses.

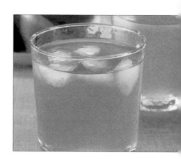

Energy 114Kcal/486kJ; Protein 1.3g; Carbohydrate 27.3g, of which sugars 27.3g; Fat 0.8g, of which saturates 0.3g; Cholesterol 0mg; Calcium 18mg; Fibre 0.3g; Sodium 7mg.

WHEATGRASS TONIC
36KCAL, 0.1G SAT FAT

Wheatgrass is grown from wheat seeds and is a concentrated source of chlorophyll and the antioxidant vitamins A, C and E. It has a distinctive, sweet flavour so this juice is blended with mild white cabbage, but it is just as tasty combined with other vegetables or fruit.

50g/2oz white cabbage
90g/3½oz wheatgrass
Serves 1

1 Cut the core from the cabbage and roughly shred the leaves. Push through a juicer with the wheatgrass (a masticating juicer is best). You could also pulse it in a food processor and push the pulp through a strainer, if you don't have a juicer.

2 Pour into a small glass and serve.

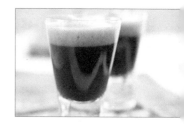

Energy 36Kcal/149kJ; Protein 3.2g; Carbohydrate 3.9g, of which sugars 3.8g; Fat 0.8g, of which saturates 0.1g; Cholesterol 0mg; Calcium 178mg; Fibre 2.9g; Sodium 130mg.

PINEAPPLE AND GINGER JUICE
120KCAL, 0.1G SAT FAT

Fresh root ginger is invigorating and has a unique flavour. In this unusual fruity blend, it is simply mixed with fresh, juicy pineapple and sweet-tasting carrot, creating a quick, easy and healthy drink that can be juiced up in minutes – and which tastes delicious too.

½ small pineapple
25g/1oz fresh root ginger
1 carrot
ice cubes
Serves 1

1 Using a sharp bread knife, cut away the skin from the pineapple, then halve it and remove the tough woody core. Roughly slice the flesh. Peel and chop the ginger, then chop the carrot.

2 Push through a juicer, or chop in a food processor and push through a strainer.

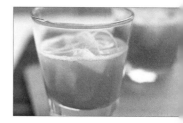

Energy 120Kcal/516kJ; Protein 1.1g; Carbohydrate 30.2g, of which sugars 29.9g; Fat 0.4g, of which saturates 0.1g; Cholesterol 0mg; Calcium 33mg; Fibre 1.2g; Sodium 33mg.

BERRY AND CHLORELLA SMOOTHIE   37KCAL, 0G SAT FAT

This berry-packed drink is positively bursting with supernutrient goodness and makes the ideal pick-me-up when energy levels are lagging. The crushed ice makes this a revitalizing beverage that is lighter than many other smoothies.

) ice cubes
50g/5oz/scant 1 cup mixed berries
  (raspberries, blackberries, redcurrants
  and blackcurrants)
)ml/4 tbsp cranberry juice
)ml/2 tsp chlorella powder
erves 1

Put the berries in a food processor or ender and add the cranberry juice.

2 Pulse until the mixture breaks down into a thick purée.

3 Add the chlorella powder to the food processor or blender and pulse again until it is mixed into the purée.

4 Finally, add the crushed ice and blend well. Pour the smoothie into a large glass and serve while it is still chilled.

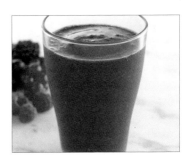

ergy 37Kcal/161kJ; Protein 2g; Carbohydrate 8g, of which sugars 8g; Fat 0g, of which saturates 0g; Cholesterol 0mg; Calcium 70mg; Fibre 5.3g; Sodium 22mg.

APRICOT AND GINGER SMOOTHIE   167KCAL, 0.6G SAT FAT

This delicious drink is packed with fibre as well as flavour, and makes a sustaining choice for a quick breakfast. It is fairly thick, so for a nger drink you could thin it down by adding some cold still or sparkling water or some more milk (the latter will add calories).

piece preserved stem ginger, plus
  15ml/1 tbsp syrup from the ginger jar
0g/2oz/¼ cup ready-to-eat dried
  apricots, halved or quartered
0g/1½oz/scant ½ cup unsweetened
  muesli (granola)
bout 200ml/7fl oz/scant 1 cup skimmed
  milk, chilled
erves 2

1 Roughly chop the preserved ginger and put it in a blender or food processor with the syrup, dried apricots, muesli and milk.

2 Process the mixture until it is smooth, adding more milk if necessary until it is of a drinkable consistency.

3 Serve immediately in wide glasses.

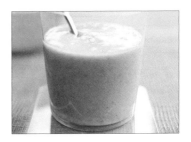

ergy 167Kcal/706kJ; Protein 6g; Carbohydrate 29.3g, of which sugars 19g; Fat 3.3g, of which saturates 0.6g; Cholesterol 0mg; Calcium 42mg; Fibre 3.1g; Sodium 65mg.

MANGO AND LIME LASSI   71KCAL, 0.4G SAT FAT

A drink and meal in one, lassis contain a useful amount of protein from the yogurt as well as nutrients from the mango. The addition of me juice helps to cut through the sweetness, but it does mean that the drink needs to be enjoyed immediately or it may curdle.

mango
nely grated rind and juice of 1 lime
5ml/1 tbsp lemon juice
lear honey, to taste
00ml/3½fl oz/scant ½ cup low-fat
  probiotic yogurt
nineral water, to dilute
extra lime, halved, to serve
erves 2

1 Peel the mango and cut away the flesh from the stone (pit). Put the flesh into a food processor or blender and add the lime rind and juice.

2 Add the lemon juice, honey to taste and yogurt and blend until smooth. Stir a little mineral water into the mixture to thin it down to the required consistency for drinking.

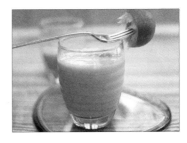

ergy 71Kcal/302kJ; Protein 3.1g; Carbohydrate 14.3g, of which sugars 14.1g; Fat 0.7g, of which saturates 0.4g; Cholesterol 1mg; Calcium 104mg; Fibre 2g; Sodium 43mg.

POPPED AMARANTH CEREAL

28KCAL, 0G SAT FAT

High in protein, B-vitamins and minerals, this grain is a nutrient-packed way to start the day. You can add some to your usual cereal or use as a delicious topping for fruit or yogurt.

20g/¾oz amaranth grain
2.5ml/½ tsp ground cinnamon
2.5ml/½ tsp clear honey
natural (plain) yogurt and/or fresh fruit,
  to serve
Serves 1

1 Heat a heavy pan over a medium heat, with the lid on. Place half the amaranth grain in the pan and shake to form a thin layer.

2 Shake the pan to ensure even distribution of heat so that the grains do not burn.

3 When the popping has stopped, after about 30 seconds, remove the pan from the heat and pour the popped amaranth into a bowl.

4 Repeat with the other half of the grain and add to the bowl. Add the cinnamon and honey and mix. Serve on top of yogurt.

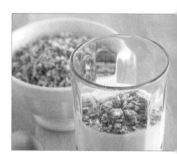

Energy 28Kcal/116kJ; Protein 0.8g; Carbohydrate 5.9g, of which sugars 1.9g; Fat 0.4g, of which saturates 0g; Cholesterol 0mg; Calcium 31mg; Fibre 0g; Sodium 2mg.

TRADITIONAL SCOTTISH PORRIDGE

115KCAL, 0G SAT FAT

Oatmeal is an excellent way to help reduce bad cholesterol in our bodies and, as it releases energy slowly, should stop you snacking mid-morning. You could substitute porridge oats or millet flakes if you like. This makes an excellent breakfast for all the family.

1 litre/1¾ pints/4 cups water
115g/4oz/1 cup pinhead oatmeal
a pinch of salt
clear honey, to taste
skimmed milk, to serve
Serves 4

1 Put the water, oatmeal and salt into a pan. Bring to the boil over a medium heat, stirring.

2 When the porridge is smooth in texture and beginning to thicken, reduce the heat to a gentle simmer.

3 Cook gently for about 25 minutes, stirring occasionally, until the oatmeal is cooked and the consistency smooth. Sweeten to taste with a small amount of honey, and serve hot with skimmed milk.

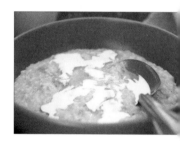

Energy 115Kcal/488kJ; Protein 3.6g; Carbohydrate 20.9g, of which sugars 0g; Fat 2.5g, of which saturates 0g; Cholesterol 0mg; Calcium 16mg; Fibre 2g; Sodium 10mg.

GRIDDLED TOMATOES ON TOAST

172KCAL, 0.9G SAT FAT

Delicious griddled tomatoes make a real treat for a weekend breakfast while on a diet, and can also be enjoyed by everyone in the family. The Parmesan cheese adds sustaining protein, as well as flavour, but you can leave it off if you prefer.

olive oil, for brushing and drizzling
6 tomatoes, thickly sliced
4 thin slices wholegrain bread
balsamic vinegar, for drizzling
salt and ground black pepper
shavings of Parmesan cheese,
  to serve (optional)
Serves 4

1 Brush a ridged griddle pan with a small amount of olive oil and heat. Lay the tomato on the pan and cook for about 4 minutes, turning once.

2 Meanwhile, toast the slices of bread. Place the tomatoes on top. Drizzle with a little olive oil and balsamic vinegar. Season and serve with shavings of Parmesan cheese.

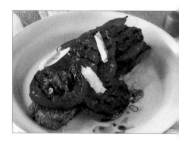

Energy 172Kcal/724kJ; Protein 3.9g; Carbohydrate 25.1g, of which sugars 5.8g; Fat 6.9g, of which saturates 0.9g; Cholesterol 0mg; Calcium 63mg; Fibre 2.3g; Sodium 171mg.

APPLE AND QUINOA BREAKFAST BARS   174KCAL, 2G SAT FAT

acked with protein, quinoa makes a nutritious addition to these delicious bars, which are perfect on mornings when time is tight and
ou need to grab something and go. They can also be enjoyed as an energy-boosting snack an hour before an aerobic session.

50ml/¼ pint/⅔ cup clear honey
0g/1½oz/3 tbsp butter
5ml/3 tbsp demerara (raw) sugar
small or 1 large eating apple,
 peeled and grated
0ml/2 tbsp puffed quinoa
0ml/2 tbsp ground flaxseeds (linseeds)
0ml/2 tbsp roughly chopped hazelnuts
.5ml/½ tsp ground cloves
ml/1 tsp mixed (apple pie) spice
0ml/2 tsp ground ginger
Makes 8

ariation Puffed quinoa is available in
any health food stores or online. If you
an't get hold of it, use twice the weight
f quinoa flakes.

1 Heat the oven to 180°C/350°F/Gas 4.
Grease a 18cm/7in square baking tin (pan),
and line with baking parchment.

2 In a large pan over low heat, heat the
honey, butter and sugar, stirring, until
the sugar has dissolved, and you have a
thin syrup.

3 Remove the pan from the heat and stir in
the remaining ingredients, until thoroughly
combined. Transfer to the prepared tin and
spread evenly into the edges with the back
of a fork.

4 Bake for 30–35 minutes until crisp at the
edges. Score into eight bars with a sharp
knife while still warm, but leave in the tin
until totally cool.

5 Wrap each one in clear film (plastic wrap)
and store in an airtight container.

Cook's tip Revered by the Incas thousands
of years ago for its stamina-increasing
powers – essential for a warrior tribe –
quinoa is a complete protein that contains
all nine essential amino acids. In addition,
it is packed with fibre along with vitamins
and minerals including iron, magnesium and
lysine, which is used for tissue repair.

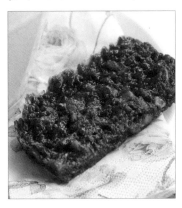

nergy 174Kcal/731kJ; Protein 2g; Carbohydrate 26g, of which sugars 22g; Fat 8g, of which saturates 2g; Cholesterol 10mg; Calcium 16mg; Fibre 1g; Sodium 35mg.

CHEWY FRUIT SLICE   110KCAL, 0G SAT FAT

Unlike conventional flapjack, these oaty bars contain only natural fruit sugars and minimal fat. They are also high in fibre and the oats
will keep you going all morning. Try to use unsulphered ready-to-eat dried apricots if you can.

75g/3oz/¾ cup ready-to-eat dried apricots,
 finely chopped
 eating apple, cored and grated
50g/5oz/1¼ cups unsweetened Swiss-style
 muesli (granola)
50ml/¼ pint/⅔ cup apple juice
5g/½oz/1 tbsp soft sunflower margarine
Makes 8

ook's tips
 Make sure the muesli (granola) is
nsweetened; many types contain high
evels of added sugar, so check the packet.
 You could use figs in place of apricots if
ou prefer; both are high in fibre.

1 Preheat the oven to 190°C/375°F/Gas 5.
Use a tiny amount of spray oil to grease a
20cm/8in non-stick sandwich tin (layer pan).

2 Mix together all of the ingredients in a
large bowl. Press the mixture into the
prepared tin and bake for 35–40 minutes,
or until the surface is until lightly browned
and firm.

3 Mark the muesli slice into eight equal
wedges with the blade of a knife and leave
to cool completely in the tin. Turn out and cut
or break along the scored lines. Store in an
airtight container.

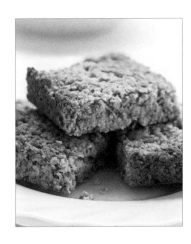

nergy 110Kcal/465kJ; Protein 2g; Carbohydrate 20g, of which sugars 12g; Fat 3g, of which saturates 0g; Cholesterol 0mg; Calcium 29mg; Fibre 3g; Sodium 86mg.

SNACKS AND LIGHT LUNCHES

PEA GUACAMOLE

103KCAL, 0.7G SAT FAT

Guacamole made with avocados is delicious and packed with goodness, but it is high in fat and calories. This fresh-tasting variation made with peas is more diet-friendly and makes a nutritious and tasty snack or light lunch served with rice cakes.

350g/12oz/3 cups frozen peas,
  completely defrosted
1 garlic clove, crushed
2 spring onions (scallions), trimmed
  and chopped
5ml/1 tsp finely grated rind and juice
  of 1 lime
2.5ml/½ tsp ground cumin
a dash of Tabasco sauce
15ml/1 tbsp extra virgin olive oil
30ml/2 tbsp roughly chopped fresh
  coriander (cilantro)
ground black pepper
a pinch of cayenne and lime slices,
  to garnish
brown rice cakes, to serve
Serves 4

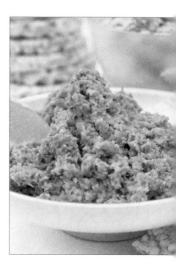

1 Put the peas, garlic, spring onions, lime rind and juice, cumin, Tabasco sauce, olive oil and ground black pepper into a food processor and process for a few minutes until smooth.

2 Add the chopped fresh coriander and process for a few more seconds until the coriander is just chopped and combined.

3 Spoon into a serving bowl, cover with clear film (plastic wrap) and chill for about 30 minutes.

4 Sprinkle over the cayenne, garnish with the lime slices and serve with some brown rice cakes.

Energy 103Kcal/425kJ; Protein 6.5g; Carbohydrate 10.4g, of which sugars 2.5g; Fat 4.3g, of which saturates 0.7g; Cholesterol 0mg; Calcium 45mg; Fibre 4.8g; Sodium 5mg.

ARTICHOKE AND CUMIN DIP

76KCAL, 0.8G SAT FAT

High in fibre and very flavoursome, artichokes can be blitzed to make a creamy dip containing many fewer calories and much less fat than hummus or other dips made with sour cream or cream cheese. Enjoy with breadsticks for a satisfying snack.

2 x 400g/14oz cans artichoke hearts
2 garlic cloves, peeled
2.5ml/½ tsp ground cumin
olive oil
ground black pepper
Serves 4

Cook's tips
• There is a large range of breadsticks available, and some are higher in fat than others. Look for plain ones, with no added salt or cheese, that have been baked with olive oil rather than any other fat.
• Using spices, such as ground cumin in this dip, means that you do not need to add salt. Lemon juice and fresh herbs also add flavour, so try replacing salt with these in other dishes too and see how they taste.

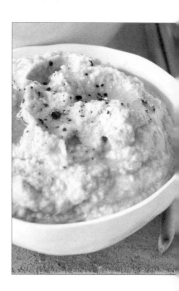

1 Drain the artichoke hearts, reserving the oil for salad dressings.

2 Put the artichoke hearts in a food processor with the garlic and ground cumin, and a generous drizzle of olive oil. Process to a smooth purée and season with black pepper to taste.

3 Spoon the purée into a serving bowl and serve with a selection of raw vegetable crudités, for dipping. When not dieting, you could drizzle a little olive oil on the top, if you like.

Variation For extra flavour, add a handful of fresh basil leaves to the artichokes before blending them in the food processor.

Energy 76Kcal/315kJ; Protein 2g; Carbohydrate 3.9g, of which sugars 2g; Fat 6g, of which saturates 0.8g; Cholesterol 0mg; Calcium 85mg; Fibre 2.7g; Sodium 121mg.

SPICED CARROT DIP

60KCAL, 0.4G SAT FAT

This delicious and unusual dip combines the sweet taste of carrots and oranges with the light spiciness of a mild curry paste. The addition of low-fat yogurt creates a creamy texture and mellows the spice flavour. Serve with crisp raw celery and cucumber sticks for dipping.

onion
carrots
grated rind and juice of 2 oranges
15ml/1 tbsp mild curry paste
150ml/¼ pint/⅔ cup low-fat probiotic yogurt
1 handful of fresh basil leaves
15–30ml/1–2 tbsp fresh lemon juice,
  to taste
Tabasco sauce, to taste (optional)
ground black pepper
celery and cucumber sticks, to serve
serves 4

Cook's tip This dip makes an ideal snack. Once prepared, divide it into portions and store in separate containers in the refrigerator, ready to take to work or grab for a quick snack. It is also delicious eaten with breadsticks or rice cakes.

1 Finely chop the onion. Peel and grate the carrots, then place the onion, carrots, orange rind and juice, together with the curry paste in a small pan. Bring to the boil, cover and simmer gently for 10 minutes, until the vegetables are tender.

2 Process the mixture in a blender or food processor until it is smooth. Leave it to cool completely.

3 Stir in the yogurt, then tear the basil leaves roughly into small pieces and stir them into the carrot mixture so that everything is well combined.

4 Add the lemon juice and Tabasco, if using, and season with pepper to taste. Chill in the refrigerator until shortly before serving.

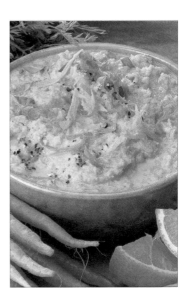

Energy 60Kcal/248kJ; Protein 2.6g; Carbohydrate 9.9g, of which sugars 9.2g; Fat 1.4g, of which saturates 0.4g; Cholesterol 1mg; Calcium 94mg; Fibre 2g; Sodium 50mg.

AUBERGINE DIP

129KCAL, 1.6G SAT FAT

Here is another tasty idea for a vegetable dip, this time made with charred aubergines flavoured with garlic, tahini, cumin, mint and lemon for a Middle Eastern taste sensation. The dip can be enjoyed with raw vegetable crudités, flatbreads, breadsticks or rice cakes.

small aubergines (eggplants)
garlic clove, crushed
60ml/4 tbsp tahini
25g/1oz/¼ cup ground almonds
juice of ½ lemon
2.5ml/½ tsp ground cumin
30ml/2 tbsp fresh mint leaves
30ml/2 tbsp olive oil
ground black pepper
serves 6

Cook's tip This is quite a calorific dip, so make sure you divide it into portions before eating it. This should be done with all snacks – it is better to measure out just one portion and then enjoy it, rather than being faced with a whole bowl and accidentally eating more than you realise.

1 Place the aubergines on the rack of a grill (broiler) pan. Grill (broil) the aubergines, turning them frequently, until the skin is blackened and blistered.

2 Remove the skin, chop the aubergine's flesh and leave it to drain in a colander. Wait for 30 minutes, then squeeze out as much liquid from the aubergines as possible.

3 Process the flesh in a blender or food processor with the garlic, tahini, almonds, lemon juice and cumin. Season with pepper, then chop half the mint and stir it in.

4 Spoon into a bowl, sprinkle the remaining mint leaves on top and drizzle with a small amount of olive oil, if you like.

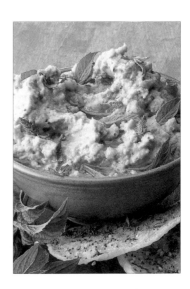

Energy 129Kcal/535kJ; Protein 3.3g; Carbohydrate 1.9g, of which sugars 1.6g; Fat 12.2g, of which saturates 1.6g; Cholesterol 0mg; Calcium 85mg; Fibre 2.5g; Sodium 4mg.

MISO BROTH WITH TOFU

71KCAL, 0.4G SAT FA

Flavoursome miso broth makes the ideal light base for a simple soup that is packed with vegetables. Tofu adds protein, makin the dish more sustaining without adding lots of fat.

1 bunch of spring onions (scallions) or
   5 baby leeks
15g/½oz fresh coriander (cilantro)
3 thin slices fresh root ginger
2 star anise
1 small dried red chilli
1.2 litres/2 pints/5 cups dashi stock or
   vegetable stock
225g/8oz pak choi (bok choy) or other Asian
   greens, thickly sliced
200g/7oz firm tofu, cut into 2.5cm/
   1in cubes
60ml/4 tbsp red miso
30–45ml/2–3 tbsp Japanese soy sauce
1 fresh red chilli, seeded and shredded
   (optional)
Serves 4

1 Cut the coarse green tops off the spring onions or baby leeks and slice the rest finely on the diagonal.

2 Place the coarse green tops in a large pan with the coriander stalks, fresh root ginger, star anise, dried chilli and dashi or vegetable stock.

3 Heat the mixture until boiling, then lower the heat and simmer for 10 minutes. Strain, return to the pan and reheat until simmering.

4 Add the green portion of the sliced spring onions or leeks to the soup with the pak choi or greens and tofu. Cook for 2 minutes.

5 Mix 45ml/3 tbsp of the miso with a little of the hot soup in a bowl, then stir it into the soup. Taste the soup and add more miso with soy sauce to taste.

6 Coarsely chop the coriander leaves and stir most of them into the soup with the white part of the spring onions or leeks. Cook for 1 minute, then ladle the soup into warmed serving bowls. Sprinkle with the remaining coriander and the fresh red chilli, if using, and serve immediately.

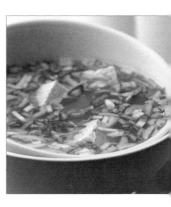

Energy 71Kcal/297kJ; Protein 7.2g; Carbohydrate 4.2g, of which sugars 3.5g; Fat 2.9g, of which saturates 0.4g; Cholesterol 0mg; Calcium 372mg; Fibre 2.6g; Sodium 884mg.

MUSHROOM SOUP

58KCAL, 1.9G SAT FA

Mushrooms have a unique, earthy flavour and make a delicious, warming and nutritious soup. Although brown cap mushrooms are listed here, you could use whichever are in season or available in a local store.

4 shallots, finely chopped
15g/½oz/1 tbsp butter
450g/1lb/6 cups brown cap (cremini)
   mushrooms, finely chopped
300ml/½ pint/1¼ cups vegetable stock
300ml/½ pint/1¼ cups semi-skimmed
   (low-fat) milk
15–30ml/1–2 tbsp chopped fresh tarragon
salt and ground black pepper, to taste
sprigs of fresh tarragon, to garnish
Serves 4

1 Peel then finely chop the shallots. Melt the butter in a large pan over a medium heat, add the shallots and cook for 5 minutes, stirring occasionally.

2 Add the mushrooms and cook gently for 3 minutes, stirring. Add the stock and milk. Bring to the boil, then cover the pan and simmer for about 20 minutes until the vegetables are soft.

3 Stir in the chopped tarragon and season to taste with salt and ground black pepper.

4 Allow the soup to cool slightly, then purée in a blender or food processor, in batches if necessary, until smooth. Return to the rinsed-out pan and reheat gently.

5 Ladle the soup into warmed soup bowls and serve with sprigs of tarragon.

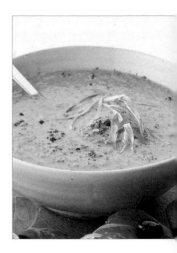

Energy 58Kcal/242kJ; Protein 3.4g; Carbohydrate 3.7g, of which sugars 3.3g; Fat 3.4g, of which saturates 1.9g; Cholesterol 8mg; Calcium 84mg; Fibre 1.4g; Sodium 44mg.

VEGETABLES IN GINGER BROTH

77KCAL, 0.2G SAT FAT

his is a great soup for using up the odds and ends of vegetables left in the chiller drawer of the refrigerator, and can be adapted to suit your references. Just make sure you use an equal amount of other vegetables, and include potatoes or other starchy vegetables to give it body.

50g/9oz/1 cup potatoes, cut into cubes
–2 fresh green chillies, sliced diagonally
50g/5oz/1 cup green beans, cut into
  2.5cm/1in lengths
50g/5oz/1 cup cabbage, shredded
ml/1 tsp salt, or to taste
0ml/2 tsp grated fresh root ginger
large garlic clove, crushed
50g/5oz/1 cup fresh spinach, washed and
  roughly chopped
5–30ml/1–2 tbsp fresh coriander (cilantro)
  leaves, chopped
ot crusty rolls, to serve (optional)
erves 4

ook's tip This soup needs to be eaten
oon after it is made since it contains
pinach and fresh herbs.

1 Put the potatoes in a medium pan, pour in 700ml/1¼ pints/3 cups water and bring to the boil. Add the chillies, reduce the heat to low, cover and cook for 7–8 minutes.

2 Add the green beans and cabbage, bring back to the boil, then cover and cook over a medium heat for 5 minutes.

3 Add the salt, ginger and garlic, replace the lid and continue to cook for 5 minutes.

4 Stir in the spinach and cook for a further 1–2 minutes, until it has wilted.

5 Add the coriander leaves, cook for about 1 minute, then remove from the heat and serve with rolls, if you like.

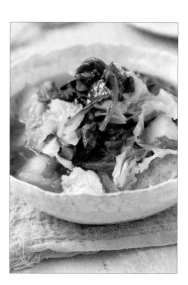

ergy 77Kcal/322kJ; Protein 3.7g; Carbohydrate 14.1g, of which sugars 4.4g; Fat 0.9g, of which saturates 0.2g; Cholesterol 0mg; Calcium 125mg; Fibre 3.7g; Sodium 66mg.

SPICY RED LENTIL SOUP

203KCAL, 0.6G SAT FAT

entils provide protein and essential nutrients and make a really sustaining, healthy soup that is a meal in itself. This fragrant spiced ersion is topped with a zingy combination of onion, parsley and lemon, but you could leave this off if time is tight.

0ml/2 tbsp olive or vegetable oil
large onion, finely chopped
garlic cloves, finely chopped
fresh red chilli, seeded and chopped
–10ml/1–2 tsp cumin seeds
–10ml/1–2 tsp coriander seeds
carrot, finely chopped
cant 5ml/1 tsp ground fenugreek
ml/1 tsp sugar
5ml/1 tbsp tomato purée (paste)
50g/9oz/generous 1 cup split red lentils
.75 litres/3 pints/7½ cups chicken stock
alt and ground black pepper

O SERVE:
small red onion, finely chopped
bunch of fresh flat leaf parsley, chopped
–6 lemon wedges
erves 4

1 Heat the oil in a heavy pan over a medium heat and stir in the onion, garlic, chilli, cumin and coriander seeds.

2 When the onion begins to colour, add the carrot and cook for 2–3 minutes. Add the fenugreek, sugar and tomato purée and lentils.

3 Pour in the stock, stir well and bring to the boil. Lower the heat, partially cover the pan with a lid and simmer for 30–40 minutes, until the lentils have broken up.

4 If the soup is too thick for your preference, thin it down to the desired consistency with a little water. Season to taste, if necessary.

5 Serve the soup as it is or whiz it in a blender until smooth, if you prefer.

6 Ladle into bowls and sprinkle with onion and parsley. Serve with lemon to squeeze over.

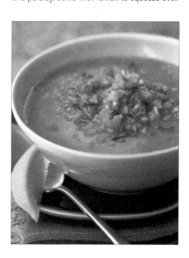

ergy 203Kcal/856kJ; Protein 11.1g; Carbohydrate 31.8g, of which sugars 7.3g; Fat 4.4g, of which saturates 0.6g; Cholesterol 0mg; Calcium 45mg; Fibre 3.5g; Sodium 26mg.

WINTER FARMHOUSE SOUP

266KCAL, 1.1G SAT FAT

Packed with starchy winter vegetables and including kidney beans and pasta, this hearty bowlful makes a wonderful low-fat lunch or supper that will provide slow-release energy for many hours after it has been eaten.

15ml/1 tbsp olive oil
1 onion, roughly chopped
3 carrots, cut into large chunks
175–200g/6–7oz turnips, cut into chunks
175g/6oz swede (rutabaga), cut into chunks
400g/14oz can chopped Italian tomatoes
15ml/1 tbsp tomato purée (paste)
5ml/1 tsp dried mixed herbs
5ml/1 tsp dried oregano
1.5 litres/2½ pints/6¼ cups vegetable stock
   or water
50g/2oz/½ cup dried macaroni or
   zero-calorie pasta
400g/14oz can red kidney beans,
   rinsed and drained
30ml/2 tbsp chopped fresh flat leaf parsley
ground black pepper
freshly grated cheese, to serve (optional)
Serves 4

Zero-calorie pasta version: 166Kcal

1 Heat the olive oil in a large pan, add the onion and cook over a low heat for about 5 minutes until softened.

2 Add the carrot, turnip and swede chunks, canned chopped tomatoes, tomato purée, dried mixed herbs and dried oregano. Stir in plenty of pepper to taste.

3 Pour in the vegetable stock or water and bring to the boil. Stir well, cover the pan, then lower the heat and simmer for about 30 minutes, stirring occasionally.

4 Add the pasta to the pan and bring to the boil over a medium heat, stirring. Lower the heat and simmer, uncovered, for about 8 minutes until the pasta is only just tender, or according to the packet instructions. Stir often to prevent the mixture sticking on the bottom of the pan.

5 Stir in the kidney beans. Heat through for 2–3 minutes, then remove the pan from the heat and stir in the parsley.

6 Taste the soup for seasoning. Serve hot in warmed soup bowls. Sprinkle with a little grated cheese if liked.

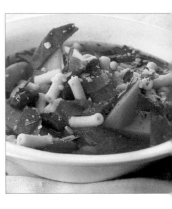

Energy 266Kcal/1118kJ; Protein 10.6g; Carbohydrate 42.3g, of which sugars 18.4g; Fat 7.2g, of which saturates 1.1g; Cholesterol 0mg; Calcium 149mg; Fibre 11.7g; Sodium 432mg.

THAI FISH SOUP

65KCAL, 0.1G SAT FAT

Meaty monkfish provides substance, flavour and texture in this fragrant soup along with high-satiety, low-fat protein. Thai ingredients such as ginger, chilli and lime juice have many health benefits, and this light broth will leave you feeling energized.

1 litre/1¾ pints/4 cups fish stock
4 lemon grass stalks
3 limes
2 small fresh hot red chillies, seeded and
   thinly sliced
2cm/¾in piece fresh root ginger, peeled and
   thinly sliced
6 coriander (cilantro) stalks, with leaves
2 kaffir lime leaves, chopped (optional)
350g/12oz monkfish fillet, skinned and
   cut into 2.5cm/1in pieces
15ml/1 tbsp rice vinegar
30ml/2 tbsp Thai fish sauce
30ml/2 tbsp chopped fresh coriander,
   to garnish
Serves 4

1 Pour the stock into a large pan and bring to the boil. Slice the bulb ends of the lemon grass diagonally into 3mm/⅛in thick pieces. Peel off four wide strips of lime rind with a vegetable peeler, avoiding the white pith. Squeeze the limes and reserve the juice.

2 Add the lemon grass, lime rind, chillies, ginger, and coriander stalks to the stock, with the kaffir lime leaves, if using. Simmer for 1–2 minutes.

3 Add the monkfish, vinegar, Thai fish sauce and half the reserved lime juice. Simmer for 3 minutes, until the fish is just tender. Although cooked, it will still hold its shape.

4 Remove the coriander stalks from the pan and discard. Taste the broth and add more lime juice if necessary. Serve the soup very hot, sprinkled with the coriander.

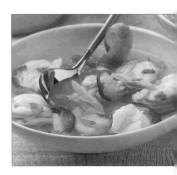

Energy 65Kcal/278kJ; Protein 14.4g; Carbohydrate 1g, of which sugars 0.8g; Fat 0.5g, of which saturates 0.1g; Cholesterol 12mg; Calcium 33mg; Fibre 0.6g; Sodium 554mg.

MUSHROOMS WITH CHILLI SAUCE 40KCAL, 0.2G SAT FAT

Mushrooms make wonderful kebabs, and their meaty texture means that they can be successfully grilled on skewers, which adds a smokey flavour that enhances their natural taste. Served with a piquant dipping sauce, this is the ideal low-fat snack or appetizer at a barbecue.

2 large field (portobello), chestnut or oyster
mushrooms or a mixture, cut in half
4 garlic cloves, coarsely chopped
6 coriander (cilantro) roots, coarsely chopped
15ml/1 tbsp sugar
30ml/2 tbsp light soy sauce
ground black pepper

FOR THE DIPPING SAUCE:
15ml/1 tbsp sugar
90ml/6 tbsp rice vinegar
5ml/1 tsp salt
1 garlic clove, crushed
1 small fresh red chilli, seeded and
finely chopped
Serves 4

Cook's tip
This dipping sauce is delicious served with
Steamed Crab Dim Sum (p39).

1 If using wooden skewers, soak eight of them in cold water for at least 30 minutes before making the kebabs. This will prevent them from burning over the barbecue or under the grill (broiler).

2 Make the dipping sauce by heating the sugar, rice vinegar and salt in a small pan, stirring occasionally until the sugar and salt have dissolved. Add the garlic and chilli, pour into a serving dish and keep warm.

3 Thread three mushroom halves on to each skewer. Lay the filled skewers side by side in a shallow dish.

4 In a mortar or spice grinder, pound or blend the garlic and coriander roots. Scrape into a bowl and mix with the sugar, soy sauce and a little pepper.

5 Brush the soy sauce mixture over the mushrooms and leave to marinate for 15 minutes. Prepare the barbecue or preheat the grill and cook the mushrooms for 2–3 minutes on each side. Serve with the dipping sauce.

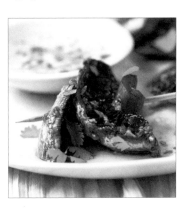

Sauce Energy 40Kcal/167kJ; Protein 3.6g; Carbohydrate 4.5g, of which sugars 4.1g; Fat 1g, of which saturates 0.2g; Cholesterol 0mg; Calcium 14mg; Fibre 2.1g; Sodium 1035mg.

BAKED CHICKPEA SAMOSAS 119KCAL, 0.8G SAT FAT

Traditional samosas are deep-fried and, though delicious, are not ideal diet fodder. In this much healthier version the samosas are baked in the oven and, containing just a few ingredients, they are very quick and easy to put together.

120ml/4fl oz/½ cup hara masala or
coriander (cilantro) sauce
275g/10oz filo pastry
2 x 400g/14oz cans chickpeas,
drained and rinsed
60ml/4 tbsp chilli and garlic oil
Serves 4

Cook's tips
• When using filo pastry you need to work quickly or it will dry out and crack. Make sure you keep any strips that you are not working with and extra pastry under a lightly dampened dish towel until required.
• Filo is much lower in fat than most other types of pastry and creates a lighter, crispier bake.

1 Preheat the oven to 220°C/425°F/Gas 7. Process half the chickpeas to a paste in a food processor.

2 Tip the puréed chickpeas into a bowl and stir in the whole chickpeas, the hara masala or coriander sauce, and a little salt if required.

3 Cut a sheet of filo pastry into three strips. Brush with a little of the flavoured oil. Place 10ml/2 tsp of the filling at one end of a strip. Turn one corner diagonally over the filling to meet the long edge. Continue folding the filling and the pastry along the length of the strip, keeping the triangular shape. Transfer to a baking sheet and repeat with the remaining filling and pastry.

4 Brush with any remaining oil and bake for 15 minutes. Serve garnished with coriander and sliced red onion.

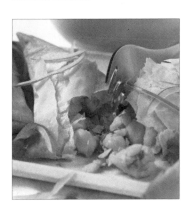

Energy 119Kcal/499kJ; Protein 4.1g; Carbohydrate 13.7g, of which sugars 0.4g; Fat 5.7g, of which saturates 0.8g; Cholesterol 0mg; Calcium 36mg; Fibre 2.2g; Sodium 99mg.

MUSSELS IN TOMATO BROTH

211KCAL, 1.2G SAT FAT

Sustainable, cheap and nutritious, mussels are extremely versatile and bring body and protein to many dishes. In this simple recipe they are served in a flavoursome tomato broth and make a delectable light meal.

1.8kg/4lb mussels in their shells
1 medium onion
1 garlic clove
30ml/2 tbsp oil
5ml/1 tsp sugar
a pinch of cayenne or chilli powder
150ml/¼ pint/⅔ cup dry (hard) cider
400g/14oz can chopped tomatoes
a small handful of chopped fresh parsley
salt and ground black pepper
Serves 4

Cook's tip It is important to clean mussels thoroughly before cooking them, or the finished dish could contain grit and sand.

1 Scrub the mussels in cold water, discarding any that have broken shells and any with open shells that do not close when given a sharp tap. Pull off the black tufts (beards) attached to the shells.

2 Peel and then finely chop both the onion and the garlic.

3 Heat the oil in a very large pan over a medium heat and add the onion, garlic and sugar. Cook, stirring occasionally, over a medium heat for about 5 minutes, or until the onion is soft and just beginning to brown. Stir in the cayenne or chilli.

4 Add the cider, tomatoes and a little seasoning and stir to combine. Bring the mixture to the boil.

5 Add the mussels, all at once. Cover tightly with a lid and cook quickly for about 5 minutes, until the shells have opened, shaking the pan occasionally.

6 Serve in warmed shallow dishes with parsley scattered over.

Cook's tip Do not be tempted to prise open and eat any mussels that have not opened up during cooking, they should be discarded

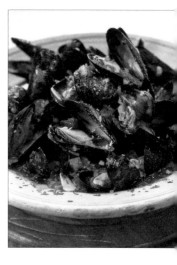

Energy 211Kcal/891kJ; Protein 21.1g; Carbohydrate 9.3g, of which sugars 4.9g; Fat 9g, of which saturates 1.2g; Cholesterol 72mg; Calcium 77mg; Fibre 1.2g; Sodium 444mg.

SUSHI-STYLE TUNA CUBES

153KCAL, 1.3G SAT FAT

Flavoursome tuna makes an ideal snack or light meal when you are working out a lot, providing lean protein that helps build muscle tone, along with brain-boosting Omega 3 oils and many other beneficial vitamins and minerals.

400g/14oz very fresh tuna, skinned
1 carton mustard and cress (optional)
20ml/4 tsp wasabi paste from a tube, or
   the same amount of wasabi powder
   mixed with 10ml/2 tsp water
60ml/4 tbsp Japanese soy sauce
8 spring onions (scallions), green part
   only, finely chopped
4 shiso leaves, cut into thin
   slivers lengthways
Serves 4

Cook's tip You really must use the freshest fish that has been specially prepared for sushi, meaning it will have been frozen in order to make it safe to eat raw.

1 Cut the tuna into 2cm/¾in cubes. If using mustard and cress, tie it into pretty bunches or arrange as a bed in four small serving bowls or plates.

2 Just 5 minutes before serving, blend the wasabi paste with the soy sauce in a bowl, then add the tuna and spring onions. Mix well and leave to marinate for 5 minutes. Do not be tempted to marinate the fish for longer, or the flesh will start to break down and 'cook'.

3 Divide the marinated fish among the bowls and add a few slivers of shiso leaves on top. Serve immediately.

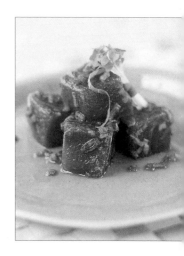

Energy 153Kcal/643kJ; Protein 24.5g; Carbohydrate 2.3g, of which sugars 2.1g; Fat 5.1g, of which saturates 1.3g; Cholesterol 29mg; Calcium 28mg; Fibre 0.4g; Sodium 806mg.

STEAMED CRAB DIM SUM

166KCAL, 1.1G SAT FAT

A traditional Cantonese dish, dim sum is intended to be enjoyed as a light snack. Many commercially produced types are laden with fat, but these tasty home-made ones are low in fat and high in flavour, as well as containing lean protein.

50g/5oz fresh white crab meat
15g/4oz minced (ground) pork
30ml/2 tbsp chopped Chinese chives
15ml/1 tbsp finely chopped red (bell) pepper
30ml/2 tbsp sweet chilli sauce
30ml/2 tbsp hoisin sauce
24 fresh dumpling wrappers
Chinese chives, to garnish
chilli oil and soy sauce, to serve
Serves 4

1 Place the crab meat, pork and chopped chives in a large bowl. Add the red pepper, sweet chilli and hoisin sauces and mix well to combine.

2 Working with 2–3 wrappers at a time (keep the rest covered), put a small spoonful of the filling mixture into the centre of each.

3 Brush the edges of each wrapper with water and fold over to form a half-moon shape. Press and pleat the edges to seal, and tap the base of each dumpling to flatten. Cover with a clean, damp cloth and make the remaining dumplings in the same way.

4 Arrange the dumplings on 1–3 oiled plates and fit inside 1–3 tiers of a bamboo steamer.

5 Cover the steamer and place over a wok of simmering water (make sure the water doesn't touch the steamer). Steam for 8–10 minutes, or until the dumplings are cooked through and become slightly translucent.

6 Divide the dumplings among four plates. Garnish with Chinese chives and serve with chilli oil and soy sauce for dipping.

Variation If you do not have a bamboo steamer, you can steam the dim sum in an electric steamer, or even in an oiled metal colander placed over simmering water.

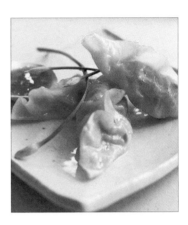

Energy 166Kcal/700kJ; Protein 14.7g; Carbohydrate 20.5g, of which sugars 1.4g; Fat 3.3g, of which saturates 1.1g; Cholesterol 46mg; Calcium 83mg; Fibre 0.8g; Sodium 287mg.

GRILLED SKEWERED CHICKEN

165KCAL, 0.8G SAT FAT

Yakitori sauce is an easy way to pack loads of flavour into dishes, and it works especially well with the grilled chicken thighs in this simple dish. Chicken thighs are slightly higher in fat than breast fillets, but they contain more nutrients.

8 chicken thighs, boned
8 large, thick spring onions
   (scallions), trimmed
lemon wedges (to serve)

FOR THE YAKITORI SAUCE:
60ml/4 tbsp sake
75ml/5 tbsp Japanese soy sauce
15ml/1 tbsp mirin
15ml/1 tbsp caster (superfine) sugar
Serves 4

1 First, make the yakitori sauce. Mix all the ingredients together in a small pan. Bring to the boil over a high heat, then reduce the heat to low and simmer for 10 minutes, or until the sauce has thickened enough to just coat the back of a spoon.

2 Cut the chicken meat into 2.5cm/1in cubes. Cut the spring onions into 2.5cm/1in-long pieces.

3 Preheat the grill (broiler) to high. Oil the wire rack to prevent sticking and spread out the chicken cubes on it.

4 Grill (broil) both sides of the chicken until the juices drip, then dip the pieces in the sauce and put them back on the rack. Grill for 30 seconds on each side, then dip in the sauce. Repeat this dipping and grilling process twice more, until the chicken is cooked.

5 Arrange the skewers on a platter and serve accompanied by lemon wedges for squeezing over.

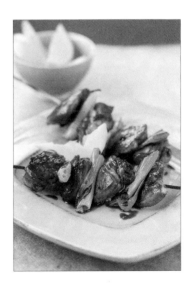

Energy 165Kcal/695kJ; Protein 22g; Carbohydrate 9g, of which sugars 8.8g; Fat 2.9g, of which saturates 0.8g; Cholesterol 105mg; Calcium 24mg; Fibre 0.4g; Sodium 1429mg.

ROASTED PEPPERS

134KCAL, 1.2G SAT FAT

The sweet, fresh taste of peppers is brought out by roasting them, and in this easy one-pot dish they are treated simply, accompanied only by tomatoes and herbs to make a colourful light lunch.

4 red or yellow (bell) peppers,
   halved and seeded
8 small or 4 medium tomatoes
15ml/1 tbsp semi-ripe sweet cicely seeds
15ml/1 tbsp fennel seeds
15ml/1 tbsp capers, rinsed
4 sweet cicely flowers, newly opened,
   stems removed
30ml/2 tbsp olive oil

FOR THE GARNISH:
a few small sweet cicely leaves
8 more flowers
Serves 4

Variation If sweet cicely is not available, you can use chervil or lovage instead.

1 Preheat the oven to 180°C/350°F/Gas 4. Place the red pepper halves in a large ovenproof dish and set aside.

2 To skin the tomatoes, cut a cross at the base, then put in a bowl and pour over boiling water. Leave to stand for 1 minute. Cut in half if they are of medium size, or leave whole if small. Place in each pepper cavity.

3 Sprinkle with sweet cicely seeds, fennel seeds and capers and about half the sweet cicely flowers. Drizzle a little olive oil all over.

4 Bake in the preheated oven for 1 hour. Serve hot, garnished with fresh sweet cicely leaves and flowers.

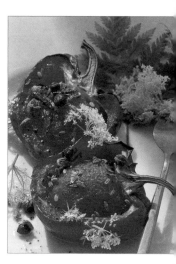

Energy 134Kcal/562kJ; Protein 4.1g; Carbohydrate 16.5g, of which sugars 16g; Fat 7.8g, of which saturates 1.2g; Cholesterol 0mg; Calcium 116mg; Fibre 6g; Sodium 29mg.

BULGUR WHEAT SALAD

149KCAL, 0.8G SAT FAT

For a sustaining lunch that will give you plenty of energy throughout the afternoon, look to salads made with grains or pulses, such as this one. Here, bulgur wheat is combined with zesty lemon juice and plenty of fresh herbs to make an appetizing bowlful.

175g/6oz/1 cup bulgur wheat,
   rinsed and drained
45ml/4 tbsp olive oil
juice of 1–2 lemons
30ml/2 tbsp tomato purée (paste)
10ml/2 tsp sugar
1 large or 2 small red onions, diced
1–2 fresh red chillies, seeded and
   finely chopped
1 bunch each of fresh mint and flat leaf
   parsley, finely chopped
salt and ground black pepper
a few fresh mint and parsley leaves,
   to garnish
Serves 6

Variation You could use cooked quinoa, couscous, rice or orzo in place of the bulgur wheat to make this sustaining salad – whichever you happen to have to hand.

1 Put the bulgur wheat into a wide bowl, pour over enough boiling water to cover it by about 2.5cm/1in, and give it a stir.

2 Cover the bowl with a plate or a pan lid and leave the bulgur wheat to steam for about 25 minutes, until it has soaked up the water and doubled in volume.

3 Pour the oil and squeeze the lemon juice over the bulgur wheat and mix.

4 Add the tomato purée and toss the mixture again until everything is combined and the bulgur wheat is well coated.

5 Add the sugar, onion, chillies, and the chopped fresh herbs. Season with salt and pepper to taste and mix well to combine. Serve at room temperature.

Variation The fresh herbs and lemon juice offset the raw onion in this dish, but you could use shallots, spring onions (scallions) or even chives if you prefer a milder flavour.

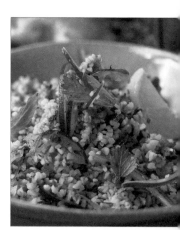

Energy 149Kcal/620kJ; Protein 3g; Carbohydrate 21.6g, of which sugars 5.4g; Fat 6.1g, of which saturates 0.8g; Cholesterol 0mg; Calcium 54mg; Fibre 1.7g; Sodium 19mg.

WARM AUBERGINE SALAD

102KCAL, 1G SAT FAT

his Turkish salad combines lots of punchy flavours and is packed with vitamins and minerals. Serve it as a dip with flatbreads or
readsticks, or you could serve it as a light lunch for two people (in which case double the nutritional information given).

tomatoes
large aubergines (eggplants), or 4 small
  thin ones
red (bell) pepper
–6 spring onions (scallions), trimmed and
  finely chopped
hot green peppers, or 1 fresh green chilli,
  seeded and finely sliced
bunch flat leaf parsley, leaves chopped
small bunch dill fronds, chopped
5ml/3 tbsp olive oil
uice of 1–2 lemons
–4 garlic cloves, crushed
alt and ground black pepper
Serves 4

Plunge the tomatoes into boiling water for
0 seconds, then refresh in cold water. Peel
way the skins. Remove the seeds and chop
he flesh.

2 Smoke the aubergines and the red pepper
directly over the gas flame, over hot charcoal
or under the grill (broiler).

3 When the skin of the pepper has buckled
and browned, plunge it immediately under
cold running water and peel off the skin.
Remove the stalk and seeds, chop the
softened flesh, and set aside.

4 When the aubergines are soft, place them
on a board and slit them open. Scoop out
the warm flesh, taking care to leave the skin
behind (this is easier if the aubergines have
been grilled over charcoal as the skin
toughens up).

5 Place the flesh in a wide bowl. Add the
pepper, spring onions, tomatoes, hot green
pepper or chilli, parsley and dill.

6 Add the olive oil, lemon juice and garlic,
and toss well. Season to taste, and serve
while still warm, with flatbreads or
breadsticks to scoop it up.

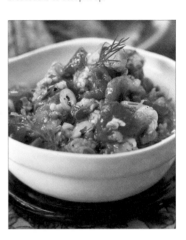

Energy 102Kcal/424kJ; Protein 3.2g; Carbohydrate 8.2g, of which sugars 7.5g; Fat 6.5g, of which saturates 1g; Cholesterol 0mg; Calcium 59mg; Fibre 4g; Sodium 14mg.

BEETROOT AND YOGURT SALAD

95KCAL, 0.6G SAT FAT

High in starch and full of antioxidants, beetroot is a versatile ingredient that pairs especially well with creamy yogurt to create a
uxurious-tasting yet low-fat salad. To save time you could use pre-cooked beetroot, but make sure they are not the pickled type.

raw beetroot (beets), washed
  and trimmed
00g/1¼lb/2¼ cups thick and creamy
  natural (plain) yogurt
garlic cloves, crushed
alt and ground black pepper
a few fresh mint leaves, shredded,
  to garnish
Serves 4

Variation To make a carrot version of this
salad, cut 4 carrots into chunks and steam
hem for about 15 minutes, until they are
ender but still retain some bite. Leave the
carrot chunks until they are cool enough to
handle, then grate and mix with the yogurt
and garlic. Season to taste.

1 Boil the beetroot in plenty of water for
35–40 minutes until tender, but not soft or
mushy. Make sure you leave the skins on
or they will 'bleed' into the water. Drain and
refresh under cold running water.

2 Wearing gloves, peel off the skins and
grate the beetroot on to a plate. Squeeze it
with your fingers to drain off excess water.
Take care not to get the juice on your clothes.

3 In a bowl, beat the yogurt with the garlic
and season with salt and pepper.

4 Add the beetroot, reserving a little to
garnish the top, and mix well. Garnish with
mint leaves.

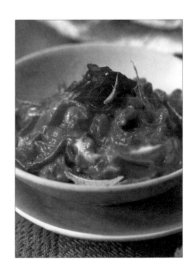

Energy 95Kcal/403kJ; Protein 7.8g; Carbohydrate 14.4g, of which sugars 13g; Fat 1.4g, of which saturates 0.6g; Cholesterol 2mg; Calcium 249mg; Fibre 1.3g; Sodium 137mg.

COURGETTE AND BEAN SALAD

183KCAL, 1.3G SAT FAT

Combining protein in the form of beans with fresh vegetables, this satisfying salad makes the perfect summer lunch while on a diet. If you want to pack it up and take it with you, omit the fresh basil, as this will blacken if left too long.

2 courgettes (zucchini), halved lengthways
   and sliced
400g/14oz can flageolet or cannellini beans,
   drained and rinsed
45ml/3 tbsp garlic-infused olive oil
grated rind and juice of 1 lemon
30ml/2 tbsp fresh basil and mint,
   roughly chopped
ground black pepper
Serves 4

Cook's tip Try to use tender young courgettes (zucchini) where possible, rather than tougher, larger, older ones. This recipe is ideal if you grow your own courgettes, as it is a quick and tasty way of using up a glut.

1 Cook the sliced courgettes in a large pan of lightly salted boiling water for 2–3 minutes, or until just tender.

2 Drain the courgettes well in a colander and refresh them under cold running water, to stop them from cooking further.

3 Transfer the drained courgettes into a bowl, add the beans and stir in the oil, lemon rind and juice and pepper, to season. Cover with clear film (plastic wrap) and chill in the refrigerator for 30 minutes, to allow the flavours to infuse.

4 Add the chopped herbs and toss together just before serving.

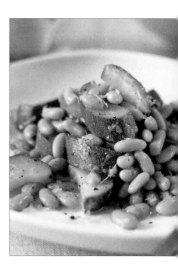

Energy 183Kcal/766kJ; Protein 7.8g; Carbohydrate 18.7g, of which sugars 4.5g; Fat 9.1g, of which saturates 1.3g; Cholesterol 0mg; Calcium 84mg; Fibre 6.7g; Sodium 391mg.

WARM SEAFOOD AND HERB SALAD

184KCAL, 1.6G SAT FAT

A decadent treat for a weekend lunch, this pretty salad is packed with protein and all the goodness of seafood. For those who are not dieting, it could be served with some fresh crusty bread to mop up the juices.

30ml/2 tbsp olive oil
15ml/1 tbsp flavoured oil, such as
   basil oil or chilli oil
finely grated rind of 1 lemon
15ml/1 tbsp lemon juice
1 garlic clove, crushed
30ml/2 tbsp chopped fresh basil
175g/6oz mixed salad leaves
225g/8oz sugar snap peas,
   sliced diagonally
400g/14oz packet frozen seafood mix,
   thawed and drained
ground black pepper
Serves 4

Cook's tip If you are using ready-cooked seafood, stir-fry it in the tiniest amount of oil for just 2 minutes to warm it through, or simply toss it in the dressing as it is and add the cold seafood to the salad.

1 Place 15ml/1 tbsp of the olive oil, the flavoured oil, grated lemon rind, lemon juice, garlic and basil in a small bowl or jug (pitcher). Season with pepper and whisk together. Set aside.

2 Place the salad leaves and sugar snap peas in a serving bowl and toss lightly to mix.

3 Heat the remaining olive oil in a large frying pan or wok, add the seafood and stir-fry over a medium heat for 5 minutes or until just cooked.

4 Arrange the warm seafood over the salad leaves, drizzle over the dressing, toss together gently to combine and serve immediately. The heat from the seafood will start to wilt the salad leaves, so do not leave it to stand before serving.

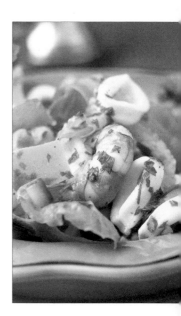

Energy 184Kcal/769kJ; Protein 18.2g; Carbohydrate 4.7g, of which sugars 3g; Fat 10.4g, of which saturates 1.6g; Cholesterol 225mg; Calcium 75mg; Fibre 2.3g; Sodium 117mg.

SEARED THAI BEEF SALAD

174KCAL, 3G SAT FAT

This delectable Thai salad requires just a little top-quality steak, which provides protein as well as a good iron hit, and makes a great high-satiety lunch that is best made in advance.

5ml/1½ tsp sunflower oil
450g/1lb fillet steak (beef tenderloin), cut into slices 2.5cm/1in thick
115g/4oz/½ cup beansprouts
1 bunch each fresh basil and mint, stalks removed, leaves shredded
1 lime, cut into slices, to serve

FOR THE DRESSING:
grated and juice (about 80ml/3fl oz) of 2 limes
30ml/2 tbsp Thai fish sauce
30ml/2 tbsp raw cane sugar
2 garlic cloves, crushed
2 lemon grass stalks, finely sliced
2 red Serrano chillies, seeded and finely sliced

Serves 6

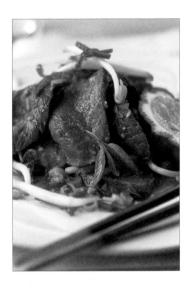

1 To make the dressing, beat the lime rind, juice, Thai fish sauce and sugar in a bowl, until the sugar dissolves. Stir in the garlic, lemon grass and chillies and set aside.

2 Pour a little oil into a heavy pan and rub it over the base with a piece of kitchen paper. Heat the pan and sear the steaks for 1–2 minutes each side. Transfer them to a board and leave to cool a little. Using a sharp knife, cut the meat into thin slices. Toss the slices in the dressing, cover and leave to marinate for 1–2 hours.

3 Drain the meat of any excess juice and transfer it to a wide serving bowl. Add the beansprouts and herbs and toss it together. Serve with lime slices to squeeze over.

Energy 174Kcal/727kJ; Protein 18.4g; Carbohydrate 7.3g, of which sugars 6g; Fat 8.1g, of which saturates 3g; Cholesterol 44mg; Calcium 28mg; Fibre 1g; Sodium 52mg.

NOODLE, TOFU AND BEAN SALAD

132KCAL, 1G SAT FAT

As nutritious as it is pretty to look at, this colourful salad includes all the food groups and makes a fabulous healthy lunch that can be packed up and taken to work, if it can be chilled once you arrive.

25g/1oz bean thread noodles
250g/9oz mixed sprouted beans
2 spring onions (scallions), shredded
75g/2oz firm tofu, diced
1 plum tomato, peeled, seeded and diced
½ cucumber, peeled and diced
30ml/2 tbsp chopped fresh coriander (cilantro)
30ml/2 tbsp chopped fresh mint
30ml/2 tbsp rice vinegar
5ml/1 tsp sesame oil
2.5ml/½ tsp chilli oil
salt

Serves 4

zero-calorie noodle version: 102Kcal

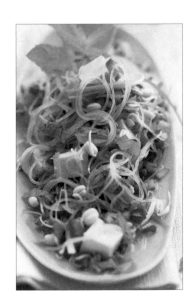

1 Place the bean thread noodles in a bowl and pour over enough boiling water to cover. Leave to soak for 12–15 minutes and then drain and refresh under cold running water and drain again. Using a pair of scissors, cut the noodles roughly into 7.5cm/3in lengths and put into a bowl.

2 Fill a wok one-third full of boiling water and place it over a high heat. Add the beans and pulses and blanch for 1 minute. Drain, transfer to the noodle bowl, and add the spring onions, tofu, tomato, cucumber and herbs.

3 Combine the rice vinegar, sugar, sesame and chilli oils and toss into the noodle mixture. Transfer to a serving dish and chill for 30 minutes before serving.

Energy 132kcal/551.76kJ; Protein 8g; Carbohydrate 17g, of which sugars 4g; Fat 4g, of which saturates 1g; Cholesterol 0mg; Calcium 112mg; Fibre 3g; Sodium 15mg.

LOW-FAT MAIN COURSES
SPANISH-STYLE VEGETABLES

185KCAL, 1.1G SAT FAT

A classic one-pot dish, roasted vegetables are so quick and easy to prepare and taste even better the next day – minimal effort for maximum healthy eating! You could vary the vegetables if you like, depending on what is in season.

2–3 courgettes (zucchini)
1 large fennel bulb
1 Spanish (Bermuda) onion
2 large red (bell) peppers
450g/1lb butternut squash
6 whole garlic cloves, unpeeled
30ml/2 tbsp olive oil
juice of 1 lemon
a pinch of cumin seeds, crushed
4 sprigs fresh thyme
4 medium tomatoes
ground black pepper
Serves 4

1 Preheat the oven to 220°C/425°F/Gas 7. Cut all the vegetables into large bitesize pieces. Smash the garlic with the flat of a knife, but leave the skins on.

2 Choose a large roasting pan into which all the vegetables will fit in one layer. Put in all the vegetables except the tomatoes.

3 Mix together the oil and lemon juice. Pour over the vegetables and toss them. Sprinkle with the cumin seeds and pepper and tuck in the thyme sprigs. Roast for 20 minutes.

4 Turn the vegetables in the oil and add the tomatoes. Cook for 15 minutes more, until tender and slightly charred around the edges.

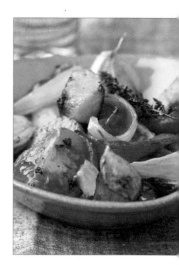

Energy 185Kcal/775kJ; Protein 6.4g; Carbohydrate 25.7g, of which sugars 19.6g; Fat 7g, of which saturates 1.1g; Cholesterol 0mg; Calcium 129mg; Fibre 9.7g; Sodium 24mg.

SPICED VEGETABLES OVER RICE

345KCAL, 1G SAT FAT

With such a high proportion of its inhabitants being vegetarian, India has a wealth of stunning vegetable dishes and the use of spices means that they are as flavoursome as they are healthy. This one makes a fabulous low-fat main course that provides lots of energy.

115g/4oz carrots, peeled and cut into
   bitesize pieces
1 small turnip, peeled and cut into
   bitesize pieces
½ small green cabbage
45ml/3 tbsp mustard oil, plus extra for
   drizzling (optional)
2.5ml/½ tsp black or brown mustard seeds
2.5ml/½ tsp cumin seeds
2 whole dried red chillies
1–2 fresh green chillies, chopped
   (seeded if preferred)
115g/4oz baby spinach leaves
2.5ml/½ tsp salt, or to taste
boiled rice, to serve
Serves 4

1 Place the carrots, turnip and cabbage in an electronic steamer, or in a steamer basket placed over a pan of simmering water, and steam until tender but firm.

2 Heat the oil in a frying pan until smoking point is reached. Switch off the heat, then add the mustard seeds followed by the cumin, dried chillies and fresh chillies.

3 Cook for 25–30 seconds, then add the steamed vegetables, spinach and salt. Stir until the spinach has wilted, then remove from the heat.

4 Put the cooked rice in individual serving dishes, spoon over the spiced vegetables and serve immediately.

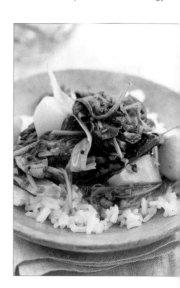

Energy 345Kcal/1452kJ; Protein 6g; Carbohydrate 55g, of which sugars 6g; Fat 13g, of which saturates 1g; Cholesterol 0mg; Calcium 109mg; Fibre 5.5g; Sodium 305mg.

BUTTER BEAN AND TOMATO STEW
138KCAL, 1.1G SAT FAT

covering all the food groups, this stew is warming enough for a cold winter's day yet light enough to be enjoyed during the summer months, when tomatoes are at their best. You could use two 400g/14oz cans of beans, although freshly cooked ones taste best.

15g/4oz/⅔ cup butter (lima) beans, soaked overnight
30ml/2 tbsp olive oil
onion, chopped
2–3 garlic cloves, crushed
25g/1oz fresh root ginger, peeled and finely chopped
pinch of saffron threads
5 cherry tomatoes
pinch of sugar
handful of fleshy black olives, pitted
ml/1 tsp ground cinnamon
ml/1 tsp paprika
small bunch of fresh flat leaf parsley
ground black pepper
Serves 4

Variation Use whichever beans you have to hand.

1 Rinse the beans and place them in a large pan with plenty of water. Bring to the boil and boil for about 10 minutes, then reduce the heat and simmer gently for 1–1½ hours until tender. Drain the beans and refresh under cold running water, then drain again.

2 Heat the olive oil in a heavy pan. Add the onion, garlic and ginger, and cook for about 10 minutes until softened but not browned. Stir in the saffron threads, followed by the cherry tomatoes and a sprinkling of sugar.

3 As the tomatoes begin to soften, stir in the butter beans. When the tomatoes have heated through, stir in the olives, ground cinnamon and paprika and warm through. Season to taste and sprinkle over the chopped parsley. Serve immediately.

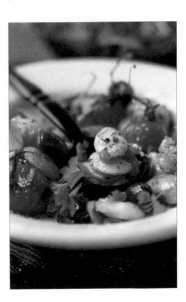

Energy 138Kcal/578kJ; Protein 5.5g; Carbohydrate 12.8g, of which sugars 3.5g; Fat 7.6g, of which saturates 1.1g; Cholesterol 0mg; Calcium 51mg; Fibre 5.2g; Sodium 605mg.

BRAISED BEANS AND LENTILS
223KCAL, 0.6G SAT FAT

High in soluble fibre and protein, this braised dish packs a real nutritional punch and keeps very well in the refrigerator if you don't use all in one meal. Dill, spring onions and lemon add zest, meaning that you don't need to include any salt.

150g/5oz/¾ cup dried mixed dried beans, soaked overnight, or two 400g/14oz cans, drained and rinsed
15g/3oz/⅔ cup brown or green lentils
15ml/1 tbsp olive oil
large onion, finely chopped
garlic cloves, crushed
5 or 6 fresh sage leaves, chopped
Juice of 1 lemon
spring onions (scallions), thinly sliced
60ml/4 tbsp chopped fresh dill
ground black pepper
Serves 4

Cook's tip Salt is not necessary in this dish, but if you feel you must use it then do not add it during the cooking time, or it will make the lentils tough. Add it at the end.

1 Put the beans, put in a large pan. Cover with cold water, bring to the boil, and cook for 1 hour. Add the lentils and cook for a further 30 minutes, until the beans and lentils are tender.

2 Drain, reserving the cooking liquid. Return the beans and lentils to the pan.

3 Heat the oil in a frying pan and fry the onion until light golden. Add the garlic and sage, cook for 30 seconds, add the mixture to the beans, then stir in the reserved liquid and simmer for 15 minutes.

4 Stir in the lemon juice and season to taste with pepper. Serve topped with a sprinkling of spring onions and dill.

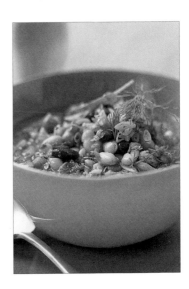

Energy 223Kcal/945kJ; Protein 14.4g; Carbohydrate 34.9g, of which sugars 5.4g; Fat 3.9g, of which saturates 0.6g; Cholesterol 0mg; Calcium 95mg; Fibre 7.9g; Sodium 13mg.

LENTILS WITH MUSHROOMS

242KCAL, 1G SAT FA

Anis is a strong flavour that pairs brilliantly with earthy mushrooms and lentils in this unusual dish. It keeps well, so why not make a big batch, divide it into portions and store in the refrigetator for evenings when you are pushed for time.

30ml/2 tbsp olive oil
1 large onion, sliced
2 garlic cloves, finely chopped
250g/9oz/3 cups brown cap (cremini)
    mushrooms, sliced
150g/5oz/generous ½ cup brown or green
    lentils, soaked overnight
4 tomatoes, cut in eighths
1 bay leaf
25g/1oz/½ cup chopped fresh parsley
30ml/2 tbsp anis spirit or anisette
salt, paprika and black pepper
Serves 4

Cook's tip If you can't find anis spirit or anisette, you could use fresh dill instead, as it has a similar flavour.

1 Heat the oil in a flameproof casserole over a medium heat. Add the onion and fry gently, with the garlic, for about 5 minutes, until softened but not browned.

2 Add the sliced mushrooms and stir to combine with the onion and garlic. Continue cooking, stirring gently, for a couple of minutes, until the mushrooms have softened.

3 Add the lentils, tomatoes and bay leaf with 175ml/6fl oz/¾ cup water. Simmer, covered, for 30–40 minutes until the lentils are soft, and the liquid has almost disappeared.

4 Stir in the parsley and anis. Season with salt, paprika and black pepper.

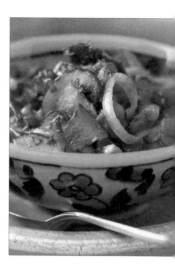

Energy 242Kcal/1018kJ; Protein 12.5g; Carbohydrate 29.8g, of which sugars 9.5g; Fat 7.2g, of which saturates 1g; Cholesterol 0mg; Calcium 83mg; Fibre 6.9g; Sodium 23mg.

DHAL

263KCAL, 1G SAT FA

This delicious lentil dish is one of the mainstays of the diet in many parts of India, and it is packed with goodness. A small amount of ghee or butter is used, which adds a lovely, authentic flavour, but you could leave it out if you prefer.

115g/4oz/½ cup red split lentils
115g/4oz/½ cup yellow split lentils
    (moong or mung dhal)
2.5ml/½ tsp ground turmeric
5ml/1 tsp salt, or to taste
25g/1oz/2 tbsp ghee or unsalted
    (sweet) butter
30ml/2 tbsp sunflower oil
2.5ml/½ tsp mustard seeds
2.5ml/½ tsp cumin seeds
2 dried red chillies, whole
2 bay leaves
1 small onion, finely chopped
30ml/2 tbsp coriander (cilantro) leaves,
    finely chopped
Serves 4

Cook's tip Adding fried spices and onions at the end of the cooking time keeps the flavours fresh and is traditional.

1 Wash both types of lentils thoroughly in a sieve (strainer) under cold water, then drain. Put them in a pan with the turmeric and add 1 litre/1¾ pints/4 cups water.

2 Bring to the boil and remove any froth with a spoon. Boil for 3–5 minutes.

3 Skim off any further froth, reduce the heat to low and cover the pan. Simmer for 30–35 minutes, then stir in the salt. Stir the lentils once or twice during cooking.

4 Heat the ghee or butter and oil in a pan over a medium heat until almost smoking. Turn the heat off and add the mustard and cumin seeds, followed by the dried chillies and bay leaves. Allow the chillies to blacken slightly, then turn the heat back up to medium.

5 Add the onion and stir-fry until the onion turns golden brown. Add all the cooked spices to the lentils and mix well.

6 Stir in the chopped coriander and remove from the heat.

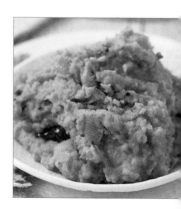

Energy 263Kcal/1110kJ; Protein 15.2g; Carbohydrate 36.6g, of which sugars 2.2g; Fat 7.4g, of which saturates 1g; Cholesterol 0mg; Calcium 49mg; Fibre 3g; Sodium 24mg.

RATATOUILLE

140KCAL, 1G SAT FAT

The perfect dish for making the most of lovely summer vegetables, ratatouille is a vibrant, healthy light dish on its own, or can be used to top zero-calorie or standard pasta or a baked potato for a more substantial meal.

2 medium aubergines (eggplants)
  (about 450g/1lb total)
60ml/4 tbsp olive oil
1 large onion, halved and sliced
2 or 3 garlic cloves, very finely chopped
1 large red or yellow (bell) pepper, seeded
  and cut into thin strips
2 large courgettes (zucchini), cut into
  1cm/½in slices
675g/1½lb ripe tomatoes, peeled, seeded
  and chopped, or 400g/14oz/2 cups canned
  chopped tomatoes
5ml/1 tsp dried herbes de Provence
salt and freshly ground black pepper

Serves 6

1 Preheat the grill (broiler). Cut the aubergine into 2cm/¾in slices, then brush the slices with oil on both sides and grill (broil) until browned, turning once. Cut into cubes.

2 Heat 15ml/1 tbsp of the olive oil in a large heavy pan or flameproof casserole and cook the onion over a medium-low heat for about 10 minutes, until lightly golden, stirring frequently.

3 Add the garlic, pepper and courgettes to the pan and cook for a further 10 minutes, stirring occasionally.

4 Add the tomatoes and aubergine cubes, dried herbs and salt and pepper and simmer gently, covered, over a low heat for about 20 minutes, stirring occasionally.

5 Uncover and continue cooking for a further 20–25 minutes, stirring occasionally, until all the vegetables are tender and the cooking liquid has thickened slightly. Serve hot or at room temperature.

Variation For a more intense flavour, roast the aubergine (eggplant), (bell) peppers and courgettes (zucchini) in 45ml/3 tbsp of the oil in an 180°C/350°F/Gas 4 oven for 20 minutes before adding to the sweated onion.

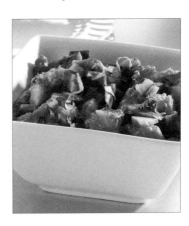

Energy 140Kcal/589kJ; Protein 8g; Carbohydrate 19g, of which sugars 10g; Fat 4g, of which saturates 1g; Cholesterol 0mg; Calcium 66mg; Fibre 6g; Sodium 536mg.

JERUSALEM ARTICHOKE STEW

147KCAL, 1G SAT FAT

This warming stew makes use of Jerusalem artichokes, which have a distinctive nutty flavour and are greatly underused in the kitchen. Combined with fresh-tasting tomatoes, herbs and lemon in this recipe, they make a nutritious change from more common vegetables.

30ml/2 tbsp olive oil
2 onions, finely chopped
2 cloves garlic, finely chopped
900g/1¼lb Jerusalem artichokes, peeled and
  cut into bitesize pieces
2 x 400g/14oz cans chopped tomatoes
10ml/2 tsp sugar
salt and ground black pepper
1 small bunch fresh coriander (cilantro),
  finely chopped, to garnish
1 lemon, cut into wedges, to serve

Serves 4

Cook's tip Jerusalem artichokes contain useful levels of vitamins and minerals as well as having a role as a prebiotic, helping to fuel the healthy bacteria in your gut.

1 Heat the oil in a heavy pan, stir in the onions and cook until they begin to colour. Add the garlic and the pieces of artichoke, and toss well to make sure they are coated in the oil.

2 Add the tomatoes to the pan, together with the sugar. Cover the pan and cook gently for 25–30 minutes, until the artichokes are tender.

3 Remove the lid and simmer the sauce over high heat to reduce it a little. Season with salt and pepper and transfer to a serving dish. Garnish with some coriander and serve with some wedges of lemon to squeeze over

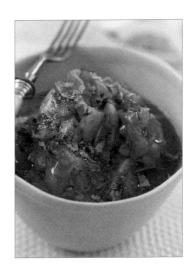

Energy 147Kcal/619kJ; Protein 3.6g; Carbohydrate 19.8g, of which sugars 17g; Fat 6.6g, of which saturates 1g; Cholesterol 0mg; Calcium 98mg; Fibre 5.1g; Sodium 97mg.

PASTA WITH ROASTED VEGETABLES   319KCAL, 1.6G SAT FA

Despite what many people think, pasta makes a very good choice when on a diet, especially if you are exercising, as it provides lots of energy with no fat. You can use zero-calorie pasta if you are cutting your calorie intake on two days per week.

1 red (bell) pepper, cut into 1cm/½in squares
1 yellow or orange (bell) pepper, cut into
    1cm/½in squares
1 aubergine (eggplant), diced
2 courgettes (zucchini), diced
75ml/5 tbsp extra virgin olive oil
15ml/1 tbsp chopped fresh flat leaf parsley
5ml/1 tsp dried oregano or marjoram
250g/9oz baby Italian plum tomatoes,
    hulled and halved lengthways
2 garlic cloves, roughly chopped
350–400g/12–14oz/3–3½ cups dried
    conchiglie or zero-calorie pasta
salt and ground black pepper
fresh marjoram or oregano flowers, to garnish
Serves 4

Zero-calorie pasta version: 176Kcal

Cook's tip Roasting brings out the natural sweetness in vegetables.

1 Preheat the oven to 190°C/375°F/Gas 5. Rinse the prepared peppers, aubergine and courgettes in a sieve (strainer) under cold running water, drain, then transfer the vegetables to a large roasting tin (pan).

2 Pour 45ml/3 tbsp of the olive oil over the vegetables and sprinkle with the fresh and dried herbs. Add salt and pepper to taste and stir well.

3 Roast the vegetables in the preheated oven for about 30 minutes, stirring two or three times.

4 Stir the halved tomatoes and chopped garlic into the vegetable mixture, then roast for 20 minutes more, stirring once or twice.

5 Meanwhile, cook the pasta according to the instructions on the packet.

6 Drain the pasta and tip it into a warmed bowl. Add the roasted vegetables and the remaining oil and toss well. Serve the pasta and vegetables hot, sprinkling each portion with a few herb flowers.

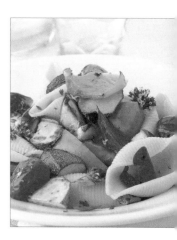

Energy 319Kcal/1343kJ; Protein 8.8g; Carbohydrate 49.6g, of which sugars 8g; Fat 10.8g, of which saturates 1.6g; Cholesterol 0mg; Calcium 34mg; Fibre 4g; Sodium 9mg.

TAGLIATELLE WITH VEG RIBBONS   348KCAL, 1.9G SAT FAT

Fresh, fast and incredibly easy, this pasta dish is perfect when you are hungry and don't want to spend ages in the kitchen. Cooking the vegetables for such a short amount of time also means they retain most of the nutritional content.

2 large courgettes (zucchini)
2 large carrots
250g/9oz fresh egg tagliatelle or pasta, or
    zero-calorie pasta
60ml/4 tbsp garlic-flavoured olive oil
ground black pepper
Serves 4

Zero-calorie pasta version: 131Kcal

Variations
• If you can't find or don't have a garlic- or herb-flavoured oil, you can use plain olive oil and simply add crushed garlic, chopped fresh herbs or chilli to it.
• Use dried pasta if you prefer.

1 Using a vegetable peeler, peel the courgettes and carrots into long ribbons.

2 Bring a large pan of water to the boil, then add the courgette and carrot ribbons. Bring the water back to the boil and cook the ribbons for 30 seconds, then drain and set aside.

3 Cook the tagliatelle or noodles according to the instructions on the packet. Drain and return to the pan. Add the vegetable ribbons, garlic-flavoured oil and pepper and toss over a medium to high heat until the pasta and vegetables are warmed through. Serve immediately.

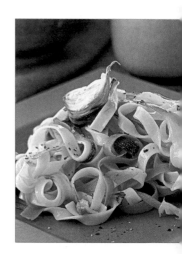

Energy 348Kcal/1464kJ; Protein 9.6g; Carbohydrate 52.1g, of which sugars 7.5g; Fat 12.7g, of which saturates 1.9g; Cholesterol 0mg; Calcium 53mg; Fibre 3.9g; Sodium 16mg

PENNE WITH VEGETABLE SAUCE

401KCAL, 0.9G SAT FAT

Leafy green vegetables are high in many vitamins and minerals and, combined with pasta, make an energizing low-fat meal that is ideal for refuelling after a hard work-out. Top with grated cheese if serving to children, to add calcium and protein.

carrots, finely diced
courgette (zucchini), finely diced
g/3oz French (green) beans
leek, washed
ripe Italian plum tomatoes
handful of fresh flat leaf parsley
ml/1 tbsp extra virgin olive oil
5ml/½ tsp sugar
5g/4oz/1 cup frozen peas
0g/12oz/3 cups dried penne
or zero-calorie pasta
ound black pepper
rves 6

ro-calorie pasta version: 163Kcals

Top and tail the French beans, then cut
em into 2cm/¾in lengths. Slice the leek.
in and dice the tomatoes. Chop the parsley.

2 Heat the oil in a medium frying pan. Add the carrots and leek. Sprinkle over the sugar and cook, stirring frequently, for 5 minutes. Stir in the courgette, French beans and peas and season with black pepper.

3 Cover the frying pan and gently cook the vegetables over a low to medium heat for 5–8 minutes, stirring from time to time, until the vegetables are just tender.

4 Meanwhile, cook the pasta in a large pan of rapidly boiling water for 10–12 minutes or according to the packet instructions if using zero-calorie water pasta, until it is tender but not soggy.

5 Drain the pasta well, return to the pan and cover to keep warm.

6 Stir in the chopped parsley and the diced chopped plum tomatoes and adjust the seasoning to taste. Toss with the pasta and serve immediately.

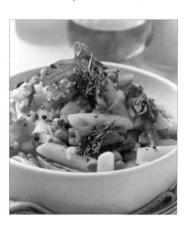

rgy 401Kcal/1698kJ; Protein 15.5g; Carbohydrate 76.7g, of which sugars 11.3g; Fat 5.7g, of which saturates 0.9g; Cholesterol 0mg; Calcium 99mg; Fibre 8.1g; Sodium 26mg.

SPRING VEGETABLE STIR-FRY

358KCAL, 1G SAT FAT

The ultimate fast food, a stir-fry is infinitely adaptable and tastes wonderful. If you want to reduce the salt further, buy reduced-salt soy sauce, and avoid using ready-made stir-fry sauces as these are often full of salt, preservatives and sugar.

ml/1 tbsp vegetable oil
ml/1 tsp toasted sesame oil
garlic clove, chopped
5cm/1in piece fresh root ginger, chopped
5g/8oz baby carrots
0g/12oz broccoli florets
5g/6oz asparagus tips
spring onions (scallions), diagonally sliced
5g/6oz/1½ cups spring greens, (collards)
finely shredded
ml/2 tbsp soy sauce
ml/1 tbsp fresh apple juice
ml/1 tbsp sesame seeds, toasted
e egg noodles or zero-calorie noodles,
to serve

rves 4

ro-calorie noodle version: 135Kcals

1 Heat a large frying pan or wok over a high heat. Add the oils and and reduce the heat. Add the garlic and sauté gently for 1 minute, stirring to prevent it burning.

2 Add the ginger, carrots, broccoli and asparagus tips to the pan and stir-fry for 4 minutes. Add the spring onions and spring greens to the pan and stir-fry for a further 2 minutes.

3 Add the soy sauce and apple juice and cook for 1–2 minutes until the vegetables are tender, adding a little water if required.

4 Spoon into four bowls and sprinkle with toasted sesame seeds. Serve with egg or zero-calorie noodles.

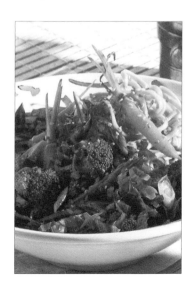

rgy 358Kcal/594kJ; Protein 7g; Carbohydrate 11g, of which sugars 10g; Fat 8g, of which saturates 1g; Cholesterol 0mg; Calcium 164mg; Fibre 3g; Sodium 571mg.

SQUASH, POTATO AND CORN STEW   329KCAL, 3.7G SAT FA

Economical and warming, this colourful stew is full of comforting flavours and sustaining ingredients. The sharp, salty tang of a little feta cheese cuts through the natural sweetness, as well as adding protein and calcium.

75ml/5 tbsp vegetable oil
1 small onion, finely chopped
2 garlic cloves, finely sliced or chopped
1 medium tomato, chopped
1 butternut squash, weighing about 1kg/
    2¼lb, peeled and cut into 2.5cm/1in
    chunks (see Cook's tip)
3 corn on the cob, cut into
    2.5cm/1in chunks
1kg/2¼lb white potatoes, peeled
    and quartered
500ml/17fl oz/generous 2 cups water
100g/3¾oz feta cheese
salt
Serves 6

1 Heat the oil in a large pan over medium heat and gently fry the onion and garlic for 10 minutes, until the onion is browned, stirring occasionally. Add the tomato and cook for another 5 minutes.

2 Add the pieces of squash, corn on the cob and potatoes to the pan and pour in the water. Season with a little salt to taste, bring to the boil and cook over medium heat for 20 minutes, covered, until the potatoes are tender.

3 Remove the pan from the heat and crumble the cheese over the vegetables. Serve immediately.

Cook's tip Peel the butternut squash with a vegetable peeler, then remove the top and bottom and chop it in half lengthways remove the seeds and cut into chunks.

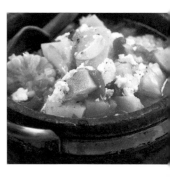

Energy 329Kcal/1382kJ; Protein 8.3g; Carbohydrate 45.2g, of which sugars 11g; Fat 14g, of which saturates 3.7g; Cholesterol 12mg; Calcium 124mg; Fibre 4.3g; Sodium 395mg

MIXED MUSHROOM STIR-FRY   238KCAL, 2G SAT FA

Mushrooms cook very quickly, making them perfect for stir-frying. Using canned and dried types, this tasty dish is a good store cupboard (pantry) standby, although you could also use any fresh ones that are available. Simply wipe them clean and cook as below.

200g/7oz canned straw mushrooms,
    drained and rinsed
200g/7oz dried Chinese mushrooms,
    soaked for 30 minutes in warm water
    until soft
200g/7oz canned button (white) or
    oyster mushrooms
30ml/2 tbsp groundnut (peanut) oil
2 slices fresh root ginger, chopped
3 garlic cloves, chopped
5ml/1 tsp cornflour (cornstarch)
30ml/2 tbsp oyster sauce
15ml/1 tbsp soy sauce
2.5ml/½ tsp ground black pepper
coriander (cilantro) leaves, to garnish
Serves 4

Cook's tip When using dried mushrooms, strain the soaking water and use 60ml/ 4 tbsp of this liquid instead of the water for blending with the cornflour (cornstarch).

1 Drain and rinse the canned mushrooms in a sieve (strainer). Cut off the hard stalks from the soaked dried mushrooms if necessary. Cut all the mushrooms into similar-sized pieces.

2 Heat the oil in a wok over a medium heat and fry the ginger and garlic for 30 seconds, or until golden brown, then add the mushrooms. Stir-fry for 2 minutes.

3 Put the cornflour into a bowl and blend with 60ml/4 tbsp water to form a smooth paste. Add the oyster sauce to the wok with the soy sauce, ground black pepper and cornflour mixture.

4 Stir and cook for 1–2 minutes, until the sauce is thick. Serve hot, garnished with coriander leaves. You could serve this with rice when not dieting.

Cook's tip Chinese dried mushrooms are available ready sliced, but these tend to b of inferior quality. Several types, such as black, straw and oyster mushrooms, are a readily available in cans.

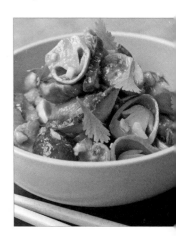

Energy 238Kcal/993kJ; Protein 8g; Carbohydrate 34g, of which sugars 1g; Fat 9g, of which saturates 2g; Cholesterol 0mg; Calcium 50mg; Fibre 0.6g; Sodium 731mg.

SPRING VEGETABLE OMELETTE — 187KCAL, 2.8G SAT FAT

Eggs, although containing some fat, are extremely nutritious and incredibly versatile. This fresh-tasting omelette makes good use of delicate-flavoured spring vegetables and provides plenty of protein along with carbohydrate from the new potatoes.

50g/2oz asparagus tips
50g/2oz spring greens (collards), shredded
15ml/1 tbsp vegetable oil
1 onion, sliced
175g/6oz cooked baby new potatoes,
 halved or diced
2 tomatoes, chopped
6 eggs
30ml/2 tbsp chopped fresh mixed herbs
ground black pepper
cherry tomatoes and leafy salad, to serve
Serves 6

1 Steam the asparagus tips and spring greens over a pan of boiling water for 8–10 minutes, until tender. Drain the vegetables and keep warm.

2 Heat the vegetable oil in a large, ovenproof frying pan over a medium heat, add the onion and cook gently for about 10 minutes until softened, stirring frequently.

3 Add the baby new potatoes to the pan and cook for 3 minutes, stirring. Gently stir in the chopped tomatoes, asparagus and greens, without breaking up the tomatoes.

4 Lightly beat the eggs in a small bowl with the herbs, and season with ground black pepper to taste.

5 Pour the beaten eggs over the vegetables, then cook over a gentle heat until the bottom of the omelette is golden brown.

6 Preheat the grill (broiler) to hot and cook the omelette under the grill for 2–3 minutes until the top is golden brown. Serve with cherry tomatoes and a salad.

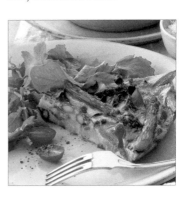

Energy 187Kcal/780kJ; Protein 11.4g; Carbohydrate 10.4g, of which sugars 3.5g; Fat 11.6g, of which saturates 2.8g; Cholesterol 285mg; Calcium 82mg; Fibre 1.8g; Sodium 118mg.

TOFU AND PEPPER KEBABS — 187KCAL, 1.6G SAT FAT

Tofu is a wonderful source of lean protein and is firm enough to hold its shape on kebabs. Interspersed with colourful peppers, these kebabs would be perfect for a barbecue while on a diet, being a much healthier alternative to a burger, steak or sausage.

250g/9oz firm tofu, rinsed and drained
50g/2oz/½ cup unsalted peanuts
2 red and 2 green (bell) peppers
60ml/4 tbsp sweet chilli dipping sauce
Serves 4

1 Pat the tofu dry on kitchen paper and then cut it into bitesize cubes. Put the peanuts in a blender or food processor and process until coarsely ground, then transfer to a plate. Turn the tofu in the ground nuts to coat the outside.

Cook's tip
Make sure you use firm tofu rather than any of the other types available. Silken tofu in particular is not suitable as it will simply fall off the skewers.
If using wooden skewers, soak them for at least 30 minutes before using.

2 If you are making the kebabs in advance, cover them with clear film (plastic wrap) and store them in the refrigerator until they are needed.

3 Preheat the grill (broiler) to moderate. Halve and seed the peppers, and cut them into large, even chunks. Thread the chunks of pepper on to four large skewers, alternating with the coated tofu cubes, and place on a foil-lined grill rack.

4 Grill (broil) the kebabs, turning frequently, for 10–12 minutes, or until the peppers and peanuts are beginning to brown. (These kebabs can also be cooked on a barbecue, if you prefer.)

5 Transfer the kebabs to plates and serve with the sweet chilli dipping sauce.

Variation If you don't like peanuts, toss the tofu cubes in sesame seeds to coat.

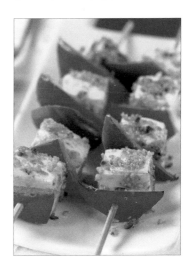

Energy 187Kcal/778kJ; Protein 10.2g; Carbohydrate 16.8g, of which sugars 15.1g; Fat 9.1g, of which saturates 1.6g; Cholesterol 0mg; Calcium 342mg; Fibre 3.7g; Sodium 214mg.

THAI SCALLOPS WITH CHILLI QUINOA   422KCAL, 2G SAT FAT

Both quinoa and scallops have many health benefits and, being high in protein, will help build lean muscle and keep you full for a long time. The fresh Thai flavours are also delicious, so this could be an ideal recipe for a special meal while on the weight-loss programme.

275g/10oz fresh scallops
3 spring onions (scallions), finely sliced
1 red (bell) pepper, finely chopped
15ml/1 tbsp sesame oil

FOR THE MARINADE:
15ml/1 tbsp sesame oil
25g/1oz fresh root ginger, grated
½ banana shallot, peeled and finely diced
5ml/1 tsp finely chopped lemon grass
5ml/1 tsp tamarind paste
45ml/3 tbsp ketjap manis (sweet soy sauce)
2 garlic cloves, crushed

FOR THE BLACK CHILLI QUINOA:
275g/10oz/1⅔ cups black quinoa
400ml/14fl oz/1⅔ cups coconut milk
600ml/1 pint/2½ cups water
½ banana shallot, finely chopped
½ fresh red chilli, finely chopped
fresh coriander (cilantro), to garnish
Serves 4

Cook's tip Health food stores are often the best place to buy more unusual types of quinoa, including the black quinoa used here.

1 First make the marinade. Place all of the ingredients into a blender and process until they form a coarse paste. Alternatively, blend them together using a mortar and pestle.

2 Place the scallops, spring onions and red pepper in a bowl and add the marinade. Cover with clear film (plastic wrap) and set aside for at least 1 hour.

3 Prepare the chilli quinoa. Rinse the quinoa in water, then transfer to a pan.

4 Add the coconut milk, water, shallot and chilli to the pan. Bring the quinoa to the boil, cover, reduce the heat and simmer for 12–14 minutes, until the quinoa is cooked but firm. Drain, reserving any excess liquid, and set aside.

5 When you are ready to serve, heat the sesame oil in a wok or large frying pan. Add the scallops, vegetables and marinade and stir-fry for 3–5 minutes on a high heat, until the scallops are cooked and fragrant, the vegetables softened and the liquid evaporated.

6 Add the black chilli quinoa to the frying pan and toss around to warm through for a couple of minutes.

7 Divide the quinoa and scallop mixture between four bowls, then pour over the warmed reserved juices from cooking the quinoa. Garnish with fresh coriander and serve immediately.

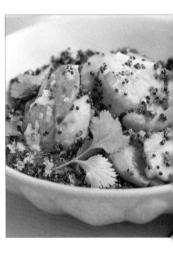

Energy 422Kcal/1742kJ; Protein 25g; Carbohydrate 55g, of which sugars 10g; Fat 12g, of which saturates 2g; Cholesterol 26mg; Calcium 138mg; Fibre 6g; Sodium 854mg.

PRAWN AND NEW POTATO STEW   218KCAL, 0.7G SAT FAT

Containing just a few simple ingredients, this is the sort of dish you can put together very quickly and then savour at leisure. Make sure you do not overcook the prawns – they have already been cooked and simply require heating through or they will become rubbery.

675g/1½lb small new potatoes, scrubbed
15ml/1 tbsp olive oil
1 garlic clove, finely chopped
400g/14oz can chopped tomatoes
300g/11oz cooked peeled prawns
   (shrimp), thawed and drained
   if frozen
15g/½oz/½ cup fresh coriander (cilantro),
   finely chopped
1 dried red chilli, crumbled
Serves 4

1 Cook the potatoes in salted boiling water for 15 minutes, until tender. Drain.

2 Heat the oil in large pan and fry the garlic for 1 minute. Pour in the tomatoes add the chilli, coriander and 90ml/6 tbsp water. Cover and simmer for 5 minutes.

3 Stir in the prawns and the potatoes and heat until just warmed through. Serve garnished with coriander and chilli.

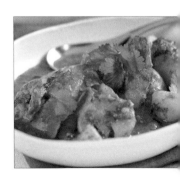

Energy 218Kcal/924kJ; Protein 16.9g; Carbohydrate 30.4g, of which sugars 5.4g; Fat 4.1g, of which saturates 0.7g; Cholesterol 146mg; Calcium 84mg; Fibre 2.9g; Sodium 171mg

PRAWN AND PEPPER KEBABS

102KCAL, 0.5G SAT FAT

These pretty sweet, hot and sour prawn kebabs pack a punch at a barbecue and are very simple to prepare. For a more sustaining meal, you could serve them with some boiled or steamed brown rice or wholemeal (whole-wheat) flatbreads and some salad.

15ml/1 tbsp pomegranate molasses
 or clear honey
15ml/1 tbsp olive oil
juice of 1 lemon
2 cloves garlic, crushed
10ml/2 tsp sugar
16 raw king prawns (jumbo shrimp),
 shelled and deveined
2 green (bell) peppers, seeded and cut into
 bitesize chunks
pinch of salt
Serves 4

1 In a bowl, mix together the pomegranate molasses, olive oil, lemon juice, garlic and sugar. Season the mixture with salt.

2 Add the prawns to the mixture, and toss gently, making sure they are all well coated with the marinade. Cover the dish and chill for 1–2 hours.

3 Prepare the barbecue, if using, or preheat a griddle or grill (broiler). Thread the prawns on to four skewers, alternating with the pepper pieces. If you are using wooden skewers, soak them for at least 30 minutes before threading them.

4 Grill (broil) the kebabs for 2–3 minutes on each side, basting them regularly with any leftover marinade while they are cooking. Serve immediately.

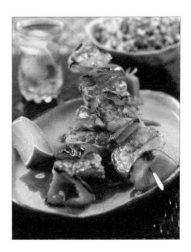

Energy 102Kcal/427kJ; Protein 9.7g; Carbohydrate 8.6g, of which sugars 8.3g; Fat 3.4g, of which saturates 0.5g; Cholesterol 98mg; Calcium 48mg; Fibre 1.4g; Sodium 109mg.

SPICY SQUID

122KCAL, 1.2G SAT FAT

Squid is a great carrier for spices and, once marinated, is very quick to cook. Ask a fishmonger to prepare the squid for you if you are not confident about doing it yourself or are short of time, or buy the frozen type and thaw it before cooking.

8 baby squid, heads, backbone and
 innards removed, and cleaned
olive oil, for brushing
a few sprigs fresh flat leaf parsley,
 roughly chopped, to garnish
1 lemon, cut into wedges, to serve

FOR THE MARINADE:
10ml/2 tsp cumin seeds, roasted
5ml/1 tsp coriander seeds, roasted
5ml/1 tsp black peppercorns
2–3 cloves garlic, crushed
grated rind of 1 lemon
15ml/1 tbsp dried sage leaves, crumbled
30ml/2 tbsp olive oil
sea salt
Serves 4

Cook's tip It is important not to overcook squid or it will quickly become rubbery and be unpleasant to eat.

1 In a mortar and pestle, pound the cumin and coriander seeds with the peppercorns. Beat in the crushed garlic, salt, lemon rind and sage leaves. Bind with the olive oil.

2 Rinse the squid well under cold running water and pat dry with kitchen paper. Using a sharp knife, sever the tentacles just above the eyes, so that the top of the head and the tentacles are joined together.

3 Using a sharp knife, score the sacs in a criss-cross pattern and rub them and the tentacles with the spicy marinade. Leave to marinate for 30 minutes.

4 Heat a griddle pan and brush with a little oil. Place the sacs and tentacles on the griddle and cook for a minute on each side. Sprinkle the parsley over the squid and serve with lemon wedges to squeeze over them.

Variation You can buy ready-prepared frozen squid, which is a useful standby ingredient to keep in the freezer. Defrost it thoroughly before using it as per the recipe.

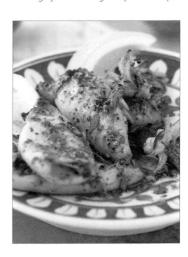

Energy 122Kcal/510kJ; Protein 13.9g; Carbohydrate 1.3g, of which sugars 0g; Fat 7.1g, of which saturates 1.2g; Cholesterol 197mg; Calcium 22mg; Fibre 0.1g; Sodium 98mg.

CEVICHE

145KCAL, 0.7G SAT FAT

The acid in the marinade gently 'cooks' the fish in ceviche, leaving the flesh succulent and tender and infused with the fresh flavour of zesy lime and the spicy kick of chilli. Accompanied by low-GI carbohydrates, this makes a sustaining and unusual main meal.

500g/1¼lb very fresh firm white fish fillets
   such as cod, halibut or coley, skinless
   and boneless
½ medium red onion, sliced lengthways
1 chilli, seeded and sliced
2 celery sticks, thinly sliced
juice of 8 limes, about 150ml/10 tbsp
4–8 lettuce leaves, to garnish
15ml/1 tbsp finely chopped parsley
salt and ground black pepper

TO ACCOMPANY:
2 medium sweet potatoes, peeled and cut
   into chunks
500g/1¼lb cassava, peeled and cut
   into chunks
1 corn on the cob
Serves 4

1 Cut the fish into bitesize pieces about 2cm/¾in across, and place in a non-metallic bowl with the onion, chilli and celery. Season with salt and pepper.

2 Pour the lime juice over the mixture and stir gently to distribute it evenly. Cover with clear film (plastic wrap) and leave to marinate for 15 minutes, then stir again and leave for another 15 minutes. The fish is ready when it has become opaque.

3 Meanwhile, boil the sweet potatoes in unsalted water for 25 minutes and boil the cassava in salted water for 20 minutes, until tender. Cut the corn on the cob into four pieces and boil in unsalted water for 10–15 minutes.

4 Arrange the lettuce leaves around the edge of a serving dish and pile the fish mixture in the middle. Serve accompanied by sweet potatoes, corn and cassava.

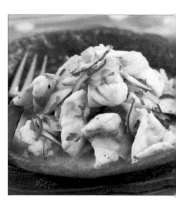

Energy 145Kcal/612kJ; Protein 18.7g; Carbohydrate 9.3g, of which sugars 8.1g; Fat 4g, of which saturates 0.7g; Cholesterol 85mg; Calcium 67mg; Fibre 1.7g; Sodium 126mg.

STEAMED RED SNAPPER

110KCAL, 0.3G SAT FAT

Attractive paper parcels of fish are as healthy as they are tasty. The fillets of fish and the fresh vegetables cook in their own juices, so that everything stays moist and succulent, the flavours are locked in and all the valuable nutrients are retained.

4 small red snapper fillets, no greater
   than 18 x 6cm/7 x 2½in, or whole
   snapper, 20cm/8in long, gutted but
   head, tail and fins intact
8 asparagus spears, hard ends discarded
4 spring onions (scallions)
60ml/4 tbsp sake
grated rind of ½ lime
½ lime, thinly sliced
5ml/1 tsp shoyu (optional)
salt
Serves 4

1 Preheat the oven to 180°C/350°F/Gas 4.

Cook's tip You can cook most types of fish using this method – just adjust the size of the baking parchment to fit the length of the fish and ensure the parcel is well sealed.

2 Cut 2.5cm/1in from the tip of the asparagus, and slice in half lengthways. Slice the asparagus stems and spring onions diagonally into thin ovals. Par-boil the tips for 1 minute in lightly salted water and drain. Set aside.

3 Cut four squares of baking parchment about 20 x 20cm/8 x 8in.

4 Place the asparagus and the spring onions in the centre of each square. Sprinkle with salt and place the fish on top. Add more salt and some sake, then sprinkle in the lime rind. Fold in two opposite corners to the centre, then the other corners, to make a loose parcel that encloses the fish. Tuck the top piece of paper under the package to secure in place.

5 Pour hot water from a kettle into a deep roasting pan fitted with a wire rack to 1cm/½in below the rack. Place the parcels on the rack. Cook in the centre of the preheated oven for 20 minutes. Check by unfolding a parcel. The fish will have changed from translucent to white.

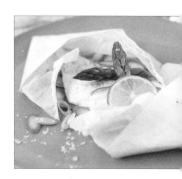

Energy 110Kcal/465kJ; Protein 20.6g; Carbohydrate 1g, of which sugars 0.9g; Fat 1.5g, of which saturates 0.3g; Cholesterol 37mg; Calcium 51mg; Fibre 0.6g; Sodium 79mg.

GRILLED TROUT

279KCAL, 2.2G SAT FAT

Trout is an oily fish that is rich in essential fatty acids, which are vital for good health. Serve this simple dish with plain boiled rice and a vegetable dish, such as steamed broccoli, for a satisfying meal.

juice of 2 lemons
cloves garlic, crushed
small trout (about 300g/11oz each),
   gutted and cleaned (you could ask a
   fishmonger to do this for you)
10ml/2 tsp zahtar
salt and ground black pepper
ground pink peppercorns
lemon, cut into wedges, to serve

Serves 6

Using a sharp knife, score the flesh of the fish diagonally three times on each side. Rub little salt and pink pepper into the fish, inside and out.

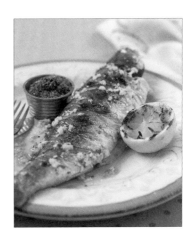

2 Prepare the barbecue or preheat a ridged griddle. In a bowl, mix together the lemon juice and crushed garlic.

3 Brush one side of the fish with the lemon juice and place it, lemon juice-side down, on an oiled rack set over the glowing coals or a high heat on the stove. Cook for around 4 minutes, then turn the fish over.

4 Brush lemon juice on the other side and cook for 4 minutes more. Transfer to a serving dish. Sprinkle the zahtar over the top and serve with lemon wedges to squeeze over the fish.

Energy 279Kcal/1176kJ; Protein 47.3g; Carbohydrate 1.7g, of which sugars 0.1g; Fat 9.4g, of which saturates 2.2g; Cholesterol 192mg; Calcium 78mg; Fibre 0.2g; Sodium 175mg.

CHINESE FISH AND TOFU STEW

238KCAL, 1G SAT FAT

Meaty monkfish holds its shape very well in stews and adds body, texture and flavour along with protein. Tofu is another form of protein and also supplies valuable calcium, while the vegetables bring both freshness and additional nutrients to the table.

350g/12oz monkfish (or similar firm-fleshed
   fish), membrane removed
dried Chinese mushrooms, soaked
   for 30 minutes in warm water
30ml/2 tbsp vegetable oil
garlic cloves, crushed
pieces of fried tofu (see Cook's Tip)
30ml/2 tbsp Chinese wine
15ml/1 tbsp hoisin sauce
30ml/2 tbsp oyster sauce
16 mangetouts (snow peas)
10ml/2 tsp cornflour (cornstarch)
salt and ground white pepper
fresh coriander (cilantro) sprigs,
   to garnish

Serves 4

Cook's tip You can buy fried tofu already prepared in cubes from most Chinese stores. The cubes are light brown and hollow inside and add flavour and protein to many Asian dishes.

1 Preheat a clay pot or flameproof casserole on the stove for a few minutes or in the oven heated to 200°C/400°F/Gas 6 for 10 minutes. Cut the fish into 2.5cm/1in chunks and slice the softened mushrooms.

2 Heat the oil in a wok over a medium heat, then add the garlic and fry for 1 minute. Add the mushrooms and fried tofu, then stir-fry for 2 minutes. Add the wine, hoisin sauce and oyster sauce and fry for 1 minute, then add 200ml/7fl oz/scant 1 cup water and bring to a simmer.

3 Add the fish and simmer gently, stirring frequently, for 2–3 minutes, or until it is just cooked. Add the mangetouts and cook for 1 minute more. Put the cornflour in a bowl and blend with 15ml/1 tbsp water, then add to the wok and cook for a few seconds until the sauce boils and thickens. Season with salt and white pepper.

4 Preheat a clay pot or flameproof casserole over a direct flame for a few minutes or in a hot oven for 10 minutes. Transfer to the clay pot and serve, garnished with coriander.

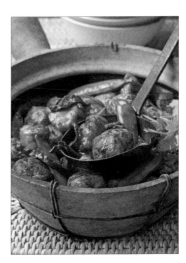

Energy 238Kcal/995kJ; Protein 20g; Carbohydrate 11g, of which sugars 2g; Fat 12g, of which saturates 1g; Cholesterol 12mg; Calcium 324mg; Fibre 0.6g; Sodium 506mg.

BAKED CITRUS FISH

129KCAL, 0.5G SAT FAT

This is such a simple dish and tastes so exquisite you will want to cook it again and again, whether for your own pleasure or for a dinner party or celebration. Steamed new potatoes make a good accompaniment, served with just the juices from the fish.

1 sea bass or grouper (weighing about
  900g/2lb), gutted and cleaned
2–3 bay leaves
1 small orange, finely sliced
1 lime, finely sliced
15ml/1 tbsp butter
salt and ground black pepper
steamed new potatoes and green
  vegetables, to serve (optional)

FOR THE MARINADE:
juice of 2 oranges
juice of 2 limes
1 clove garlic, crushed
Serves 4

1 Whisk together all the ingredients for the marinade. Place the fish in a dish and pour the marinade over it. Cover with clear film (plastic wrap) and chill for 1–2 hours. Preheat the oven to 180°C/ 350°F/Gas 4.

2 Transfer the fish to an ovenproof dish and spoon the marinade over it. Tuck the bay leaves under it and arrange several slices of orange and lime alternately along the inside, and on top of the fish.

3 Cover the dish with foil and bake for 15 minutes. Remove the foil, dot the fish with butter and bake uncovered for a further 10 minutes. Serve immediately, with new potatoes and green vegetables if you like.

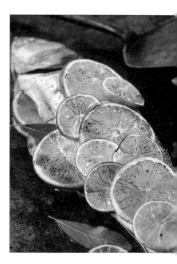

Energy 129Kcal/543kJ; Protein 24.3g; Carbohydrate 0.9g, of which sugars 0.7g; Fat 3.2g, of which saturates 0.5g; Cholesterol 100mg; Calcium 164mg; Fibre 0.1g; Sodium 87mg.

TAMARIND FISH STEW

317KCAL, 0.1G SAT FAT

Tamarind is a common ingredient in Asian cooking and acts as a souring agent that cuts through the richness of fish and gives the dish a lovely depth of both flavour and colour. If you can't find it, use the juice from a lemon instead, although it is not quite the same.

115g/4oz/1 cup dried tamarind pulp,
  soaked in 350ml/12fl oz/1½ cups water
  for 20 minutes
1kg/2¼lb fish steaks, such as sea
  bream, grouper or sea bass
15–30ml/1–2 tbsp olive oil
1 onion, halved and sliced
4 cloves garlic, chopped
5ml/1 tsp cumin seeds
10ml/2 tsp ground turmeric
5ml/1 tsp ground fenugreek
2.5ml/½ tsp chilli powder
12 small new potatoes, peeled
1 x 400g/14oz can of plum tomatoes,
  drained of juice
5ml/1 tsp palm sugar or light muscovado
  (brown) sugar
salt and ground black pepper
1 bunch coriander (cilantro), chopped
Serves 6

1 Squeeze the tamarind pulp in your hand to separate the pulp from the seeds and stalks, then strain the pulp through a sieve (strainer). Reserve the strained pulp and liquid.

2 Heat the oil in a heavy pan and sear the fish steaks for 1–2 minutes on each side, then transfer them to a plate. Stir the onion, chilli, garlic and cumin seeds into the pan and cook until they begin to colour. Add the spices to the pan, then toss in the potatoes and cook for 2–3 minutes. Stir in the tomatoes and add the sugar.

3 Pour the tamarind water into the pan and bring the liquid to the boil. Reduce the heat, cover the pan, and simmer gently for about 15 minutes, until the potatoes are tender.

4 When the potatoes are cooked, season with salt and pepper to taste, then slip in the seared fish steaks. Cover the pan again and cook gently for 10 minutes, until the fish is cooked. Stir half the coriander into the stew and garnish with the rest. Serve immediately.

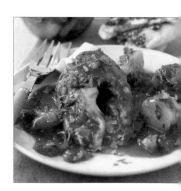

Energy 317Kcal/1337kJ; Protein 32g; Carbohydrate 26g, of which sugars 5g; Fat 10g, of which saturates 1g; Cholesterol 63mg; Calcium 103mg; Fibre 1.2g; Sodium 291mg.

THAI FISH CURRY

172KCAL, 1.7G SAT FAT

Oil-rich fish such as salmon contain omega-3 fatty acids that promote good health, and they should be eaten regularly – at least once a week. The robust flesh stands up well to the strong Asian flavours in this delicous, aromatic curry.

350g/12oz salmon fillet
500ml/17fl oz/2¼ cups vegetable
   stock
4 shallots, finely chopped
2 garlic cloves, finely chopped
2.5cm/1in piece fresh galangal,
   finely chopped
1 lemon grass stalk, finely chopped
2.5ml/½ tsp dried chilli flakes
15ml/1 tbsp Thai fish sauce
5ml/1 tsp palm sugar or light muscovado
   (brown) sugar
boiled rice, to serve (optional)
Serves 4

1 Place the salmon in the freezer and leave for 30–40 minutes to firm up the flesh. Remove and discard the skin, then use a sharp knife to cut the fish into 2.5cm/1in cubes, removing any stray bones with your fingers or with tweezers as you do so.

2 Pour the stock into a large, heavy pan and bring it to the boil over a medium heat. Add the shallots, garlic, galangal, lemon grass, chilli flakes, fish sauce and sugar. Bring back to the boil, stir well, then reduce the heat and simmer gently for 15 minutes to reduce slightly and intensify the flavours.

3 Add the fish, bring back to the boil, then turn off the heat. Leave to stand for 10–15 minutes until cooked through.

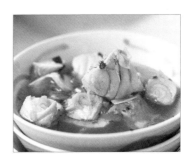

Energy 172Kcal/717kJ; Protein 18.2g; Carbohydrate 3.2g, of which sugars 2.5g; Fat 9.7g, of which saturates 1.7g; Cholesterol 44mg; Calcium 24mg; Fibre 0.3g; Sodium 307mg.

COD, TOMATO AND PEPPER STEW

312KCAL, 1.2G SAT FAT

Really fresh cod fillets have a sweet, delicate flavour and pure white flaky flesh that is delicous in this stew, but you must make sure it is sourced responsibly, or use an alternative such as pollack or coley.

450g/1lb potatoes, cut into thin slices
20ml/4 tsp olive oil
1 red onion, chopped
1 garlic clove, crushed
1 red (bell) pepper, seeded and diced
1 yellow (bell) pepper, seeded and diced
225g/8oz mushrooms, sliced
one 400g/14oz and one 225g/8oz can
   chopped tomatoes
150ml/¼ pint/⅔ cup dry white wine
450g/1lb skinless, boneless cod fillet,
   cut into 2cm/¾in cubes
50g/2oz/½ cup pitted black olives,
   roughly chopped
15ml/1 tbsp chopped fresh basil
15ml/1 tbsp chopped fresh oregano
salt and ground black pepper
fresh oregano sprigs, to garnish
cooked courgettes (zucchini), to serve
Serves 4

Cook's tip If making this dish for children, use fish stock instead of white wine.

1 Preheat the oven to 200°C/400°F/Gas 6. Par-boil the potatoes in a pan of lightly salted, boiling water for 4 minutes. Drain thoroughly, then add 5ml/1 tsp of the oil and toss together to mix. Set aside.

2 Heat the remaining oil in a large frying pan, add the onion, garlic and red and yellow peppers and cook for 5 minutes, stirring occasionally.

3 Stir in the mushrooms, tomatoes and white wine, bring to the boil and boil rapidly for a few minutes, stirring frequently, until the sauce has reduced slightly.

4 Add the fish, olives, herbs and seasoning to the tomato mixture.

5 Spoon the mixture into a lightly greased casserole or ovenproof dish and arrange the potato slices over the top, covering the fish mixture completely.

6 Bake, uncovered, for about 45 minutes until the fish is cooked and tender and the potato topping is browned. Garnish with fresh oregano sprigs and serve with the cooked courgettes.

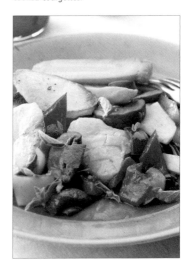

Energy 312Kcal/1312kJ; Protein 26.3g; Carbohydrate 32.4g, of which sugars 14.1g; Fat 6.7g, of which saturates 1.2g; Cholesterol 89mg; Calcium 77mg; Fibre 7.5g; Sodium 385mg.

TURKEY AND CORN STEW

269KCAL, 1.2G SAT FAT

Turkey is a great lean source of protein and makes a good alternative to ubiquitous chicken breast fillets. The sweetness of the corn is offset by the kick from the fresh chilli purée and, accompanied by brown rice, this makes a sustaining meal.

6 corn cobs
30ml/2 tbsp vegetable oil
500g/1¼lb skinless turkey breast fillet,
    cut into 2cm/¾in cubes
1 medium onion, finely chopped
2 garlic cloves, sliced or crushed
2 red chillies, seeded and blended to a
    purée in 60ml/4 tbsp water
500ml/17fl oz/generous 2 cups chicken
    or vegetable stock
salt
chopped parsley, to garnish
cooked brown rice, to serve
Serves 4

1 Slice off the corn kernels from the cob. Blend them to a smooth purée in batches.

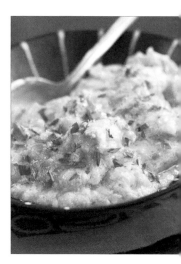

2 Heat the oil in a large pan and fry the turkey over a high heat for 8–10 minutes, until golden on all sides.

3 Stir in the onion and garlic, reduce the heat slightly and cook for about 10 minutes, stirring frequently, until the onion is caramelized and brown.

4 Add the chilli purée and cook for 3 minutes, then pour in the stock. Bring to the boil and simmer for 20 minutes. Season to taste.

5 Add the puréed corn and simmer for a further 15 minutes, until thick. Garnish with parsley and serve the turkey stew with cooked brown rice.

Energy 269Kcal/1132kJ; Protein 33.8g; Carbohydrate 16.2g, of which sugars 4g; Fat 8.1g, of which saturates 1.2g; Cholesterol 71mg; Calcium 19mg; Fibre 2.2g; Sodium 269mg.

TURKEY PATTIES

146KCAL, 0.6G SAT FAT

Containing hardly any fat, these turkey patties are a slimmer's dream when it comes to burgers and will solve all your problems if you are invited to a barbecue while you are on the diet. They are also a family-friendly treat that will go down well at any time.

675g/1½lb minced (ground) turkey
1 small red onion, finely chopped
grated rind and juice of 1 lime
a small handful of fresh thyme leaves
15ml/1 tbsp olive oil
salt and ground black pepper
bread rolls and salad leaves, to serve
Serves 6

Variations
• Minced (ground) chicken or pork could be used instead of turkey in these burgers.
• You could also try chopped oregano, parsley or basil in place of the thyme, and lemon rind instead of lime.

Cook's tip These patties freeze really well. Simply shape the raw mixture then create a pile, placing a sheet of greaseproof (waxed) paper between each pattie, and freeze.

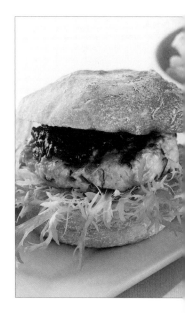

1 Mix together the turkey, onion, lime rind and juice, thyme and seasoning in a large bowl, using a spoon or your hands.

2 Cover with clear film (plastic wrap) and chill in the refrigerator for up to 4 hours. Dampen your hands, then divide the mixture into six equal portions and shape into round patties.

3 Preheat a griddle pan. Brush the patties with a little oil, then place them on the pan and cook for 10–12 minutes. Turn the patties over, brush with more oil and cook for 10–12 minutes on the second side, or until cooked through.

4 Slice the rolls in half, place some salad leaves on the bottom half and top with the burger and the other half of the roll.

Energy 146Kcal/615kJ; Protein 27.8g; Carbohydrate 2.4g, of which sugars 1.4g; Fat 2.9g, of which saturates 0.6g; Cholesterol 64mg; Calcium 27mg; Fibre 0.5g; Sodium 58mg.

DRY-FRIED HOT-AND-SOUR CHICKEN   389KCAL, 2G SAT FAT

hicken thighs contain more minerals than white meat and, sliced into thin strips, cook just as quickly. They are also more flavoursome
nd can stand up to the intense taste of the Chinese aromatics and ingredients that accompany the meat in this dish.

50g/1lb boneless chicken thigh fillets
5ml/1 tbsp groundnut (peanut) oil
5g/1oz fresh root ginger, sliced into strips
Chinese or English celery sticks, sliced
spring onions (scallions), sliced into
  short lengths
0ml/2 tbsp chilli bean paste
5ml/½ tsp caster (superfine) sugar
5ml/½ tsp Sichuan peppercorns, crushed
5ml/1 tbsp rice vinegar
oodles or zero-calorie noodles, to serve
erves 4

ero-calorie noodle version: 166Kcal

ook's tip Do not use more chilli bean
aste than specified as it is high in salt and
an overpower the dish.

1 Cut the chicken into strips about 2cm/¾in
wide. Heat the oil in a wok and fry the
ginger for 1 minute, or until golden brown.

2 Add the chicken, celery, spring onions and
chilli bean paste. Stir-fry for 2 minutes over a
medium heat.

3 Add the sugar to the wok, then the
peppercorns and wine, and continue to
stir-fry for a further 2 minutes, or until the
chicken is nearly cooked through.

4 Sprinkle 30ml/2 tbsp water over the
chicken and cook until the wok is nearly
dry and the chicken is cooked through and
has a darkish hue from the sauce. Serve
immediately with noodles.

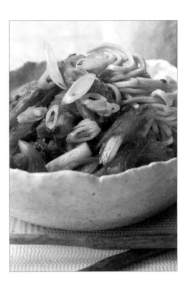

nergy 389Kcal/729kJ; Protein 24g; Carbohydrate 4g, of which sugars 3g; Fat 7g, of which saturates 2g; Cholesterol 118mg; Calcium 25mg; Fibre 0.3g; Sodium 308mg.

CHICKEN ON PITTA   408KCAL, 2.1G SAT FAT

Marinading chicken tenderizes the flesh and adds flavour, meaning little or no salt is required. This Middle Eastern-inspired sandwich
nakes a sustaining main meal and will be enjoyed by all the family.

skinless chicken breast fillets
alt and ground black pepper
pitta breads, tahini sauce and pickled
  vegetables, to serve

OR THE MARINADE:
0ml/3 tbsp olive oil
uice of 2–3 lemons
0ml/2 tsp white wine or cider vinegar
cloves garlic, crushed
cinnamon stick, broken into pieces
rated rind of ½ orange
–6 cardamom pods, crushed
erves 4

ook's tip Wholemeal (whole-wheat) pitta
s the best choice as it is higher in fibre and
as a lower GI than white types, meaning
: will keep you fuller for longer.

1 Mix together the ingredients for the
marinade in a large bowl and then toss
the chicken breast fillets in the mixture.
Cover and chill for at least 6 hours.

2 Preheat the oven to 180°C/350°F/Gas 4.
Put the chicken in an ovenproof dish and
bake for 20 minutes, basting with the
marinade several times during the cooking.

3 When cooked, lift the chicken out, shred,
and return to the dish with any remaining
marinade, season and return to the oven for
10 minutes.

4 Warm the pitta breads in the oven for
5 minutes. Serve the chicken with the pitta,
accompanied by a tahini sauce and some
pickled vegetables.

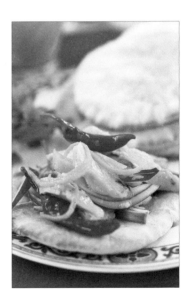

nergy 408Kcal/1726kJ; Protein 40.2g; Carbohydrate 44.7g, of which sugars 1.8g; Fat 8.9g, of which saturates 2.1g; Cholesterol 65mg; Calcium 90mg; Fibre 1.7g; Sodium 499mg.

INDIAN CHICKEN STEW

308KCAL, 1G SAT FA

This lightly spiced stew includes rice along with vegetables and meat, making it a one-pot wonder that everyone can enjoy. Adjust the amount of chilli used according to taste; keeping the seeds in will make it hotter.

1 chicken, weighing about 1.5kg/3lb 5oz
7.5ml/1½ tsp salt, or to taste
8 large garlic cloves, crushed
15g/½oz fresh root ginger, finely chopped
1 large onion, finely chopped
2 bay leaves
450g/1lb small potatoes, peeled
225g/8oz carrots, cut at an angle
150g/5oz/1¼ cups cooked basmati rice
3–4 fresh green chillies, slit open
    lengthways (seeded if preferred)
fine strips of fresh root ginger and
    tomatoes, to garnish
Serves 4

Cook's tip When preparing chillies, wear gloves or wash you hands immediately after.

1 Joint the chicken, remove the skin and trim off any excess fat. Alternatively, ask a butcher to do this for you or buy pre-jointed breast, thigh and drumstick pieces.

2 Put the prepared chicken into a large pan with a lid and pour in 550ml/18fl oz/2½ cups cold water.

3 Add the salt, garlic, ginger, onion, and bay leaves. Bring to the boil, reduce the heat, cover and cook for 10 minutes.

4 Add the potatoes, cover with the lid and cook for 20 minutes. Add the carrots, cover and cook for about 10 minutes, until they are just tender.

5 Add the cooked rice and green chillies, simmer for 5–6 minutes, then remove from the heat. Ladle into bowls and garnish with strips of ginger and tomato.

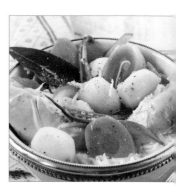

Energy 308Kcal/1303kJ; Protein 37g; Carbohydrate 32g, of which sugars 7g; Fat 4g, of which saturates 1g; Cholesterol 135mg; Calcium 49mg; Fibre 2.9; Sodium 729mg.

CHICKEN CASSEROLE WITH ONIONS

282KCAL, 0.6G SAT FA

The health benefits of onions have been recognized for thousands of years and they are at their most effective when eaten raw, as in this recipe, in which they are marinated and served with a simple chicken casserole.

1 chicken, about 1kg/2lb in weight
1.2 litres/2 pints/5 cups water
2 onions, quartered
2 carrots, peeled and each cut into thirds
2 cloves garlic, smashed in their skins
4–5 cloves
3–4 cardamom pods
250g/8oz spinach leaves, washed
salt and ground black pepper
flat bread, to serve

FOR THE MARINATED ONIONS:
2 onions, halved and sliced
seeds of half a pomegranate
30ml/2 tbsp white wine vinegar
Serves 4

Variations If you don't like pickled onion, you could cook them in a tiny amount of olive oil until just soft and then serve.

1 Place the onions and pomegranate seeds in a bowl and toss in the vinegar. Cover and set aside to marinate.

2 Place the chicken in a deep pan and cover with water. Add the onions, carrots, garlic, cloves, cardamom pods and seasoning.

3 Bring the water in the pot to the boil then reduce the heat, cover, and simmer for about 25 minutes.

4 Lift the chicken out of the pan and check the seasoning of the stock. If it lacks flavour, boil rapidly for 10 minutes to reduce.

5 Skin the chicken, cut it into joints, and return to the stock to heat through along with the spinach leaves.

6 Serve the chicken in shallow bowls, spooning the carrots and spinach leaves over it. Top each bowl with a spoonful of the marinated onions and pomegranate seeds, and serve with bread.

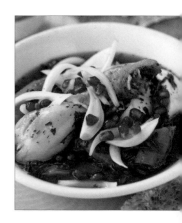

Energy 282Kcal/1188kJ; Protein 46.2g; Carbohydrate 19g, of which sugars 15.3g; Fat 2.9g, of which saturates 0.6g; Cholesterol 123mg; Calcium 163mg; Fibre 6.9g; Sodium 204mg.

THAI PORK STIR-FRY

174KCAL, 1.2G SAT FAT

lean pork fillet is much lower in fat than many cuts of pork and cooks very quickly, making it a good choice for a stir-fry. Adding flour eates an unctuous, thick sauce in this recipe, which makes good use of store cupboard staples.

50g/1lb lean pork fillet (tenderloin)
0ml/2 tbsp plain (all-purpose) flour
ml/1 tsp sunflower oil
onion, roughly chopped
garlic clove, crushed
green (bell) pepper, seeded and sliced
50g/12oz carrots, cut into thin strips
25g/8oz can bamboo shoots, drained
5ml/1 tbsp white wine vinegar
5ml/1 tbsp soft brown sugar
0ml/2 tsp tomato purée (paste)
0ml/2 tbsp light soy sauce
alt and ground black pepper
erves 4

Thinly slice the pork. Season the flour and ss the pork in it to coat.

2 Heat the oil in a large frying pan or a wok and cook the pork for 5 minutes, until golden. Remove the pork and drain on kitchen paper. You may need to do this in several batches.

3 Add the onion and garlic to the pan and cook for 3 minutes. Add the pepper and carrots and stir-fry over a high heat for 6–8 minutes, or until beginning to soften slightly.

4 Return the meat to the pan with the bamboo shoots. Add the remaining ingredients with 120ml/4fl oz/½ cup water and bring to the boil. Simmer for 2–3 minutes, or until piping hot. Adjust the seasoning, if necessary, and serve immediately.

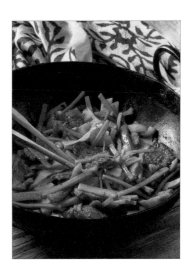

nergy 174Kcal/729kJ; Protein 24g; Carbohydrate 4g, of which sugars 3g; Fat 7g, of which saturates 2g; Cholesterol 118mg; Calcium 25mg; Fibre 0.3g; Sodium 308mg.

PORK MEATBALLS WITH PASTA

408KCAL, 2.1G SAT FAT

firm family favourite, meatballs can easily be made in advance and chilled in the refrigerator or frozen until required. The addition of ek and mushrooms in these makes them lighter and more nutritious and bulks them out without adding fat.

50g/1lb lean minced (ground) pork
leek, finely chopped
15g/4oz mushrooms, finely chopped
5ml/1 tbsp chopped fresh thyme
5ml/1 tbsp tomato purée (paste)
egg, beaten
0ml/2 tbsp plain (all-purpose) flour
5ml/1 tbsp sunflower oil
50–500g/12oz–1¼lb pasta or
zero-calorie pasta
esh thyme sprigs, to garnish

OR THE TOMATO SAUCE:
garlic clove, crushed
00g/14oz can chopped tomatoes
5ml/1 tbsp chopped fresh basil
alt and ground black pepper
erves 4

ero-calorie noodle version: 295Kcal

1 To make the meatballs, stir together the pork, leek, mushrooms, thyme, tomato purée, egg and flour. Shape into balls, cover and chill.

2 Place all the sauce ingredients in a pan, season to taste, then bring to the boil. Boil, uncovered, for 10 minutes, until thickened.

3 Preheat the oven to 180°C/350°F/Gas 4. Heat the oil in a frying pan, add the meatballs and cook in batches until lightly browned all over. Place in a shallow, ovenproof dish and pour the tomato sauce over. Cover and bake for about 1 hour until cooked through.

4 Meanwhile, cook the pasta according to the packet instructions until al dente. Drain and place in bowls, spoon the meatballs and sauce over the top and serve garnished with thyme.

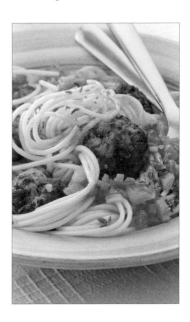

nergy 408Kcal/1726kJ; Protein 40.2g; Carbohydrate 44.7g, of which sugars 1.8g; Fat 8.9g, of which saturates 2.1g; Cholesterol 65mg; Calcium 90mg; Fibre 1.7g; Sodium 499mg.

FRIED RICE WITH BEEF

232KCAL, 2.7G SAT FAT

You may have thought that a recipe with this title could never be included in a diet, but in fact since just a small amount of oil is used it is actually low in fat and, containing rice, protein and vegetables, it is a very well balanced dish that covers all the food groups.

200g/7oz lean beef steak, trimmed and cut
   into very thin strips
5ml/1 tsp sunflower oil
2 garlic cloves, finely chopped
1 egg
250g/9oz/2¼ cups cooked rice
½ medium head broccoli, coarsely chopped
30ml/2 tbsp dark soy sauce
15ml/1 tbsp light soy sauce
5ml/1 tsp palm sugar or light muscovado
   (brown) sugar
15ml/1 tbsp Thai fish sauce
ground black pepper
chilli sauce, to serve
Serves 4

1 Heat the oil in a wok or frying pan and cook the garlic over a low to medium heat until golden. Do not let it burn. Increase the heat to high, add the steak and stir-fry for 2 minutes.

2 Move the pieces of beef to the edges of the wok or pan and break the egg into the centre. When the egg starts to set, stir-fry it with the meat.

3 Add the rice and toss everything together, scraping up any residue on the base, then add the broccoli, soy sauces, sugar and fish sauce and stir-fry for 2 minutes more. Season with pepper and serve immediately with chilli sauce.

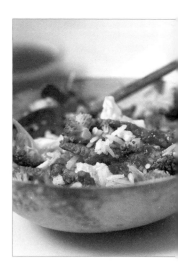

Energy 232Kcal/975kJ; Protein 16.9g; Carbohydrate 24.5g, of which sugars 5g; Fat 8.1g, of which saturates 2.7g; Cholesterol 77mg; Calcium 52mg; Fibre 1.4g; Sodium 321mg.

BULGUR WHEAT WITH LAMB

366KCAL, 2.5G SAT FAT

This is another complete meal in a bowl, and the secret to its low-fat status lies in the fact that only a small amount of meat is used, the bulk of the dish being supplied by bulgur wheat and nutrition-packed chickpeas.

15ml/1 tbsp olive oil
1 onion, finely chopped
5ml/1 tsp ground cumin
5ml/1 tsp ground fenugreek
200g/7oz lean lamb, cut into chunks
200g/7oz/1⅓ cups cooked chickpeas
250g/9oz/1½ cups coarse bulgur wheat
salt and ground black pepper
1 small bunch fresh coriander (cilantro),
   finely chopped, to garnish
Serves 6

Cook's tip When not on a diet, use 15ml/
1 tbsp ghee instead of oil, for added flavour.

1 Rinse and drain the bulgur wheat. Heat the olive oil in a heavy pan and add the chopped onion. Cook, stirring, until the onion softens and begins to turn a golden brown colour.

2 Stir the ground cumin and fenugreek into the onions, and stir through until they release their aromas.

3 Toss the chunks of lamb into the pan and stir to coat the meat in the cooked onion and spices.

4 Add about 900ml/1½ pints/3¾ cups water to the pan and bring it to the boil. Season with salt and pepper and stir gently. Reduce the heat and simmer for 20 minutes.

5 When all the water has been absorbed, turn off the heat, cover the pan with a dish towel, followed by the lid, and leave the bulgur wheat to steam for a further 10 minutes. Do not lift the lid during this time or you will affect the cooking.

6 Fork through the mixture to separate the grains, then transfer the bulgur wheat and lamb mixture into a warmed serving dish and garnish with the chopped coriander. Serve immediately.

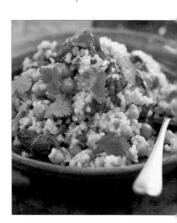

Energy 366Kcal/1533kJ; Protein 18.5g; Carbohydrate 51.8g, of which sugars 2.7g; Fat 10.3g, of which saturates 2.5g; Cholesterol 25mg; Calcium 87mg; Fibre 4g; Sodium 46mg.

IVE-SPICE BEEF IN BEAN SAUCE 399KCAL, 2.7G SAT FAT

 favourite take-away (take-out) dish, this home-made version is much lower in fat, calories and salt than ones you have delivered and
astes so much better. Check the label on the chilli bean paste and try to buy the one that is lowest in salt.

50g/1lb sirloin or rump (round) steak,
 trimmed of fat
ml/1 tsp cornflour (cornstarch)
0ml/2 tbsp sesame oil
5ml/1 tbsp dark soy sauce
0ml/2 tbsp groundnut (peanut) oil
 garlic cloves, crushed
5g/1oz fresh root ginger, peeled and
 finely chopped
 spring onions (scallions), cut into
 5cm/2in lengths
5ml/1 tbsp chilli bean paste
.5ml/½ tsp five-spice powder
.5ml/½ tsp caster (superfine) sugar
hick egg noodles or zero-calorie noodles,
 to serve
hredded spring onions, to garnish
erves 4

ero-calorie noodle version: 261Kcal

1 Slice the beef into thin strips about
1cm/½in thick, then put them into a bowl.

2 Put the cornflour into a small bowl and
blend in the sesame oil and soy sauce.
Sprinkle this mixture over the beef and toss
to coat. Leave to marinate for 10 minutes.

3 Heat the groundnut oil in a wok and fry
the garlic and ginger for 30 seconds, or until
light brown. Toss in the beef and stir-fry over
a high heat for 1 minute.

4 Add the onions, chilli bean paste, five-spice
powder, sugar and 45ml/3 tbsp water.

5 Stir the beef and sauce over a high heat
for 2 minutes, or until the sauce is thick.
Serve immediately, with noodles, sprinkled
with shredded spring onions.

Cook's tip Don't be tempted to use a
ready-made sauce – these tend to be high
in calories, fat and salt and also rarely taste
as good as one you have made yourself.

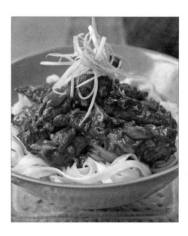

nergy 399Kcal/745kJ; Protein 27g; Carbohydrate 43.4g, of which sugars 1.6g; Fat 9.3g, of which saturates 2.7g; Cholesterol 103mg; Calcium 21mg; Fibre 2g; Sodium 161mg.

3EEF AND MUSHROOM BURGERS 211KCAL, 2G SAT FAT

ulking out burgers with breadcrumbs and mushrooms reduces their fat and calorie content considerably as well as giving them a
utritional boost. Using very lean beef makes them a waist-friendly choice too, and they taste wonderful.

 small onion, chopped
50g/5oz/2 cups mushrooms
50g/1lb very lean minced (ground) beef
0g/2oz/1 cup fresh wholemeal
 (whole-wheat) breadcrumbs
ml/1 tsp dried mixed herbs
5ml/1 tbsp tomato purée (paste)
our, for shaping
alt and ground black pepper
urger buns or pitta bread, sliced gherkins,
 red onion rings and salad leaves
erves 4

ook's tip The mixture is quite soft, so
andle it carefully and use a fish slice or
hetal spatula for turning to prevent the
urgers from breaking up during cooking.

1 Place the onion and mushrooms in a food
processor and process until finely chopped.

2 Add the beef, breadcrumbs, herbs, tomato
purée and seasonings. Process for a few
seconds, until the mixture binds together but
still has some texture.

3 Divide the mixture into four pieces, then
press them into burger shapes using lightly
floured hands.

4 Cook the burgers in a large non-stick
frying pan, or under a hot grill (broiler), for
12–15 minutes, turning once, until evenly
cooked. Serve in burger buns or pitta bread
with gherkins, onions rings and salad leaves.

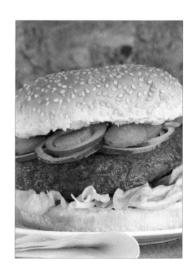

nergy 211Kcal/889kJ; Protein 28.1g; Carbohydrate 13.4g, of which sugars 3g; Fat 5.4g, of which saturates 2g; Cholesterol 65mg; Calcium 38mg; Fibre 1.8g; Sodium 178mg.

DESSERTS AND HEALTHY SWEET TREATS

TROPICAL-SCENTED FRUIT SALAD 87KCAL, 0G SAT FAT

Oranges and strawberries are both great sources of vitamin C, and the passion fruit adds an intense exotic fragrance, as well as further vitamin value and fibre in this pretty salad. Try to buy strawberries in season or at least make sure they are ripe.

400g/14oz/3½ cups strawberries, hulled
  and halved
4 oranges, peeled and segmented
2 passion fruits
120ml/4fl oz/½ cup fresh, chilled tropical
  fruit juice
Serves 4

1 Put the hulled and halved strawberries and peeled and segmented oranges into a bowl.

2 Halve the passion fruit and using a teaspoon scoop the flesh into the bowl.

3 Pour the tropical fruit juice over the fruit and toss gently. Cover and chill in the refrigerator or serve immediately.

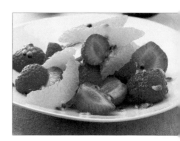

Energy 87Kcal/371kJ; Protein 2.4g; Carbohydrate 20g, of which sugars 20g; Fat 0.3g, of which saturates 0g; Cholesterol 0mg; Calcium 78mg; Fibre 3.5g; Sodium 14mg.

PAPAYA, LIME AND GINGER SALAD 55KCAL, 0.2G SAT FAT

This refreshing, fruity salad makes a lovely light dessert, and it is perfect for the summer months. Choose really ripe, fragrant papayas for the best flavour. Papaya is a very nutritious fruit with good antioxidant value provided by vitamins A and C.

2 large ripe papayas
juice of 1 fresh lime
2 pieces preserved stem ginger, finely sliced
Serves 4

Variation This refreshing fruit salad is delicious made with other tropical fruit. Try using 2 ripe, peeled, stoned (pitted) mangoes in place of the papayas.

1 Cut the papayas in half lengthways and scoop out the seeds, using a teaspoon. Using a sharp knife, thickly slice the flesh and arrange on a platter.

2 Squeeze the lime juice over the slices of papaya and sprinkle them with the finely sliced stem ginger. Serve the fruit salad immediately or chill.

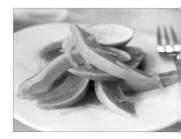

Energy 55Kcal/234kJ; Protein 0.8g; Carbohydrate 13.4g, of which sugars 13.4g; Fat 0.2g, of which saturates 0g; Cholesterol 0mg; Calcium 36mg; Fibre 3.3g; Sodium 8mg.

ORANGE GRANITA WITH STRAWBERRIES 79KCAL, 0G SAT FAT

A granita is a refreshing alternative to ice cream, and makes the ideal dessert while on a diet. The combination of orange juice in the granita and the accompanying portion of fresh, ripe strawberries provides a generous amount of vitamin C.

6 large juicy oranges, squeezed
350g/12oz ripe strawberries, halved,
  to serve
finely pared strips of orange rind,
  to decorate
Serves 4

1 Pour the freshly squeezed orange juice into a shallow freezerproof bowl. Place in the freezer. After 30 minutes, beat with a wooden spoon. Repeat at 30-minute intervals over a 4-hour period.

2 Serve the granita with strips of orange rind and the strawberries.

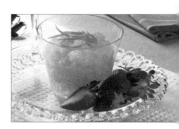

Energy 79Kcal/336kJ; Protein 2.4g; Carbohydrate 18g, of which sugars 18g; Fat 0.2g, of which saturates 0g; Cholesterol 0mg; Calcium 85mg; Fibre 3.5g; Sodium 13mg.

APRICOT AND GINGER COMPOTE 181KCAL, 1G SAT FAT

esh ginger adds warmth to this stimulating dish and complements the flavour of the juicy apricots. Dried apricots provide a
ncentrated source of valuable vitamins and minerals, making this a great choice for a healthy dessert or even breakfast.

0g/12oz/1½ cups dried (preferably
unsulphured) apricots
m/1½in piece fresh root ginger,
finely chopped
0g/7oz/scant 1 cup low-fat natural (plain)
probiotic yogurt
rves 4

ok's tips
Ready-to-eat dried fruit doesn't require
aking overnight, but does contain
eservatives, unlike the unsulphured type.
Fresh ginger freezes really well. Peel the
ot, divide it into portions and store them
a plastic bag in the freezer.

1 Cover the apricots with boiling water, then
leave to soak overnight.

2 Place the apricots and their soaking water
in a pan, add the fresh root ginger and bring
to the boil.

3 Reduce the heat to low and simmer for
10 minutes until the fruit is soft and plump
and the water becomes syrupy.

4 Strain the apricots over a bowl, reserving
the syrup, and discard the ginger. Serve
warm with the reserved syrup and a
spoonful of yogurt.

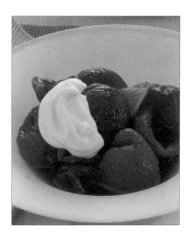

ergy 181Kcal/772kJ; Protein 6g; Carbohydrate 37g, of which sugars 36g; Fat 2g, of which saturates 1g; Cholesterol 6mg; Calcium 165mg; Fibre 16g; Sodium 53g.

OACHED PUMPKIN 157KCAL, 0G SAT FAT

e sweet orange flesh of pumpkin appears in many guises, from soups and purées to pies and, in this case, desserts. Here it is lightly
ached in a simple sugar syrup and makes a nutritious sweet finale to a meal when you feel in need of a sugar hit.

0g/1lb/2¼ cups sugar
5ml/8fl oz/1 cup water
ce of 1 lemon
cloves
g/2¼lb peeled and seeded pumpkin flesh,
cut into roughly same-size cubes
or rectangular blocks
eam or crème fraîche, to serve (optional)
rves 6

riation You could try other squash if you
e – butternut works particularly well.

ok's tip Although desserts are lovely,
ey are often high in sugar and fat and
ould be reserved for the occasional treat.
y to wait at least 15 minutes after
ishing a main course before eating
ssert, as this gives your body time to
tablish how full it really is. You will often
d that the sweet craving will pass and
u no longer want anything else.

1 Put the sugar and water into a deep, wide
heavy pan. Bring the liquid to the boil over a
medium heat, stirring all the time, until the
sugar has dissolved.

2 Boil the sugar syrup gently for 2–3 minutes,
then reduce the heat and stir in the lemon
juice and the cloves.

3 Add the pumpkin pieces to the pan and
bring the liquid back to the boil.

4 Reduce the heat, put the lid on the pan,
and poach the pumpkin gently, turning the
pieces over from time to time, until they are
tender and gleaming. Depending on the size
of your pieces, this may take 45 minutes to
1 hour.

5 Leave the pumpkin to cool in the pan, then
lift the pieces out of the syrup and place
them in a serving dish.

6 Spoon most, or all, of the syrup over
the pumpkin pieces and serve at room
temperature, or chilled with cream or crème
fraîche if you like.

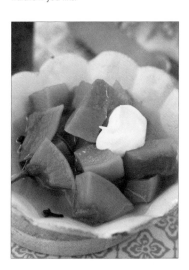

ergy 157Kcal/671kJ; Protein 1.2g; Carbohydrate 41.7g, of which sugars 40.8g; Fat 0.3g, of which saturates 0g; Cholesterol 0mg; Calcium 69mg; Fibre 2.2g; Sodium 12mg.

FLAXSEED QUINOA MUFFINS

287KCAL, 3G SAT FAT

These tasty muffins contain useful amounts of protein in the form of quinoa, which means they make you feel fuller for longer. They are an ideal snack for eating about 2 hours before a rigorous aerobic workout, or can be enjoyed for breakfast on the go.

250ml/8fl oz/1 cup buttermilk
150ml/¼ pint/⅔ cup vegetable oil
2 eggs
175g/6oz/1½ cups quinoa flour
115g/4oz/1 cup ground flaxseeds (linseeds)
5ml/1 tsp baking powder
5ml/1 tsp ground cinnamon
5ml/1 tsp ground nutmeg
115g/4oz/⅔ cup caster (superfine) sugar
50g/2oz/⅓ cup raisins
30ml/2 tbsp whole flaxseeds, for sprinkling
Makes 12

1 Preheat the oven to 200°C/400°F/Gas 6. Mix together the buttermilk, oil and eggs.

2 Sift the flour into a large bowl, then stir in the ground flaxseeds, baking powder, ground cinnamon, nutmeg, sugar and raisins.

3 Make a well in the centre of the dry ingredients, then pour in the buttermilk and egg mixture, stirring briefly to just combine the ingredients. The mixture needs to be of a dropping consistency to ensure a soft crumb, so add a little extra buttermilk if required.

4 Divide the mixture between 12 muffin tins (pans), lined with paper cases if you wish.

5 Sprinkle the top of each muffin with a few whole flaxseeds, and use the end of a teaspoon to push any exposed raisins into the batter if you want to avoid any scorching as they cook.

6 Bake for 18–20 minutes, until the muffins are well risen and firm to the touch. Remove from the tins and cool on a wire rack.

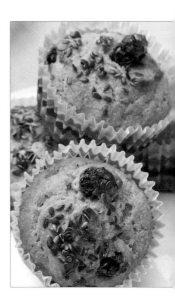

Energy 287Kcal/1197kJ; Protein 6g; Carbohydrate 25g, of which sugars 14g; Fat 19g, of which saturates 3g; Cholesterol 23mg; Calcium 51mg; Fibre 2g; Sodium 24mg.

ORANGE OATIES

110KCAL, 0G SAT FAT

These easy-to-make low-fat cookies are so delicious that it is difficult to believe that they are healthy too. As they are packed with flavour and wonderfully crunchy the whole family will love them.

175g/6oz/¾ cup clear honey
120ml/4fl oz/½ cup orange juice
90g/3½oz/1 cup rolled oats, toasted
115g/4oz/1 cup plain (all-purpose) flour
115g/4oz/generous ½ cup golden caster
    (superfine) sugar
finely grated rind of 1 orange
5ml/1 tsp bicarbonate of soda
    (baking soda)
Makes 16

Cook's tip Take care not to overcook these oaties as they burn easily.

1 Preheat the oven to 180°C/350°F/ Gas 4. Line two baking sheets with baking parchment.

2 Put the honey and orange juice in a small pan and simmer over a low heat for 8–10 minutes, stirring occasionally, until the mixture is thick and syrupy.

3 Put the oats, flour, sugar and orange rind into a bowl.

4 Mix the bicarbonate of soda with 15ml/ 1 tbsp boiling water and add to the flour mixture, together with the honey and orange syrup. Mix well with a spoon.

5 Place spoonfuls of the mixture on to the prepared baking sheets, spaced slightly apart, and bake for 10–12 minutes, or until golden brown.

6 Leave to cool on the baking sheets for 5 minutes before transferring to a wire rack to cool completely.

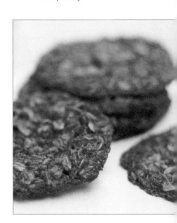

Energy 110Kcal/466kJ; Protein 1.5g; Carbohydrate 26.2g, of which sugars 16.6g; Fat 0.6g, of which saturates 0g; Cholesterol 0mg; Calcium 18mg; Fibre 0.6g; Sodium 4mg.

DATE SLICE

198KCAL, 1G SAT FAT

emon-flavoured icing tops these scrumptious, low-fat bars, which are full of succulent fruit and crunchy seeds – the perfect mid-
norning pick-me-up with a cup of coffee or tea.

75g/6oz/¾ cup light muscovado
 (brown) sugar
75g/6oz/1 cup ready-to-eat dried
 dates, chopped
15g/4oz/1 cup self-raising (self-rising) flour
0g/2oz/½ cup unsweetened Swiss
 muesli (granola)
0ml/2 tbsp sunflower seeds
5ml/1 tbsp poppy seeds
0ml/2 tbsp sultanas (golden raisins)
 or raisins
50ml/¼ pint/⅔ cup plain (natural)
 low-fat yogurt
egg, beaten
00g/7oz/1¾ cups icing (confectioners')
 sugar, sifted
mon juice
5–30ml/1–2 tbsp pumpkin seeds
lakes 16

1 Preheat the oven to 180°C/350°F/Gas 4.
Line a 28 x 18cm/11 x 7in shallow baking
tin (pan) with baking parchment.

2 In a large mixing bowl, stir together all the
ingredients, except the icing sugar, lemon
juice and pumpkin seeds.

3 Spread the mixture in the prepared baking
tin and bake for about 25 minutes, until the
surface is golden brown. Leave to cool.

4 To make the topping, put the icing sugar
in a bowl and stir in just enough lemon juice
to make a spreading consistency. Spread the
icing over the baked date mixture and
sprinkle generously with pumpkin seeds.
Leave to set before cutting into squares
or bars.

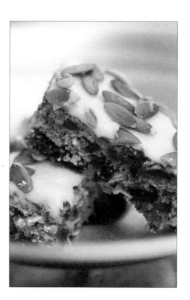

ergy 198Kcal/839kJ; Protein 3g; Carbohydrate 42g, of which sugars 35g; Fat 3g, of which saturates 1g; Cholesterol 15mg; Calcium 72mg; Fibre 2g; Sodium 46mg.

CAROB AND CHERRY COOKIES

112KCAL, 3G SAT FAT

implicity itself to make, these little cookies are given a chocolate-like flavour by the addition of carob and are deliciously crisp and
runchy. They make a great alternative to a standard cookie when you get a chocolate craving.

0g/3½oz/7 tbsp unsalted butter, at room
 temperature, diced
5g/3oz/scant ½ cup caster
 (superfine) sugar
5g/3oz/⅓ cup light muscovado
 (brown) sugar
egg
50g/5oz/1¼ cups self-raising
 (self-rising) flour
5g/1oz/2 tbsp carob powder
0g/2oz/¼ cup glacé (candied) cherries,
 quartered
0g/2oz carob bar, chopped
lakes 20

ook's tip Carob is usually available in
ealth food stores and in the wholefoods
ctions of larger supermarkets.

1 Preheat the oven to 180°C/350°F/Gas 4.
Line two large baking sheets with pieces of
baking parchment.

2 Put the unsalted butter, caster sugar,
muscovado sugar and the egg in a large
mixing bowl and beat well together until
the mixture is smooth and creamy.

3 Add the flour, carob powder, cherries and
chopped carob bar to the mixture and mix
well with a wooden spoon until thoroughly
combined, making sure the carob powder is
completely blended in.

4 Shape the mixture into walnut-size balls
and place, spaced slightly apart to allow for
spreading, on the prepared baking sheets.

5 Bake for about 15 minutes. Leave on the
baking sheets for about 5 minutes before
transferring to a wire rack to cool.

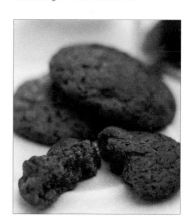

ergy 112Kcal/474kJ; Protein 1g; Carbohydrate 17g, of which sugars 11g; Fat 5g, of which saturates 3g; Cholesterol 22mg; Calcium 38mg; Fibre 0g; Sodium 35mg.

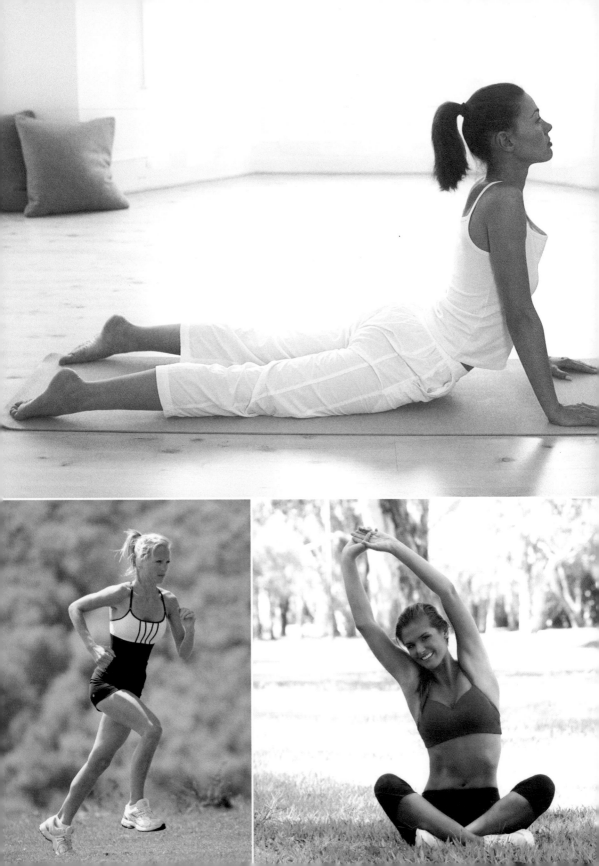

GET MOVING!

This section is all about exercise. Before you start, you need to assess how fit – or unfit – you are as well as determine your body shape and weight, and this chapter contains all the information you need to do this. There then follows an exercise section – which is split into two halves, each with a warm-up and a cool-down – starting with aerobic exercises and then moving on to strengthening and toning.

HEALTH AND FITNESS

Fitness is the key to a healthy mind and body. It is based on stamina, strength and suppleness – with better shape and self-esteem as well as improved long-term health as the bonuses. Being fit also makes you feel good overall and more able to take on new challenges in other aspects of life.

Most of us know that if we were fitter, we would probably have more confidence and a greater zest for life. But although we are more health-conscious about our diet nowadays, regular exercise is still not a part of many people's daily lives. Surveys always draw the same conclusions as to the reasons for this: lack of time, energy, interest and confidence. However, getting fit – and getting a better body – is neither as difficult nor as time-consuming as it may appear to be, and you will probably enjoy it.

HOW FIT DO YOU NEED TO BE?

There is no such thing as standard fitness – it depends on your make-up and why you want to be fit: being able to run a marathon, for example, is different from honing stamina, strength and suppleness to improve physical shape and overall health. For exercise to be of any help, it should boost your metabolism and improve your cardiovascular (heart and circulation) and respiratory (breathing) systems.

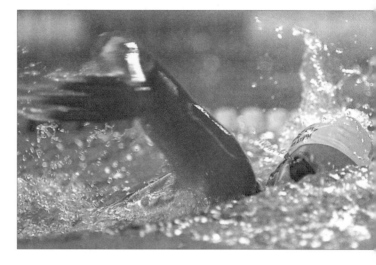

MAKING GOALS AND RECORDING YOUR RESULTS

Finding a goal that will inspire you is one of the secrets of success. To achieve that goal, you must have a motive that is important enough to give you an iron will, such as improving your figure for a special event (for example, your wedding and honeymoon), buying

Above Regular swimming sessions are a very effective way of keeping the whole body in good physical condition.

yourself a longed-for figure-hugging dress, or simply boosting your fitness levels generally. Set the 21-day deadline and stick to it. Depending on what you want to achieve, a three-week plan is ideal because it is not too long and if you persevere (take it week by week or day by day – whichever you find easiest), you will soon see results. However, be realistic: if your goals are too high you are more likely to fail; if they are too low, you will not have enough of a challenge.

Goals will inspire you, but speedy results are the key to keeping up regular exercise – it is perfectly natural that you will want to see rewards for all your hard work – although it is advisable to build up a pattern gradually.

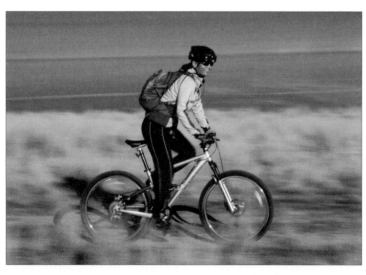

Left Being fit and healthy will enable you to get out and about and exercise in different locations – whether running, walking, cycling or taking part in adventure activities.

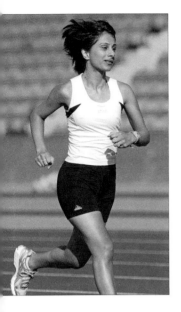

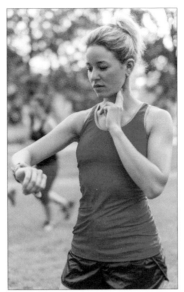

Far left Running is one of the cheapest and most accessible forms of exercise, which burns off a considerable number of calories.
Left Taking your pulse is a way of assessing how fit you are and if you are exercising hard enough to impact on your fitness.

certain range. The list below outlines the ideal exercise heart-rate ranges for different age groups:

Age	Pulse Range
20+	130–160
30+	124–152
40+	117–144

To find out your active pulse rate per minute, rest two fingers lightly on your pulse immediately after exercising, count the beats for 10 seconds and multiply by 6.

CAUTIONS

Before taking up any form of rigorous exercise or training, you should consult your doctor – especially if any of the following conditions apply to you:

- Diabetes or epilepsy
- Over 35 years of age with a long history of inactivity
- Cardiovascular or respiratory issues
- Chronic joint or back problems
- Obesity
- Pregnancy
- Heavy drinking or smoking

The amount of exercise you need to do to improve your fitness and lose weight is 30 minutes' aerobic activity five times a week. This means bouts of exercise vigorous enough to make you fairly breathless (but not gasping for breath), ideally followed by at least 10 minutes' stretching and toning. Doing toning and stretching on your 'rest' days will really maximize results. If you are unfit, this may seem daunting, but power-walking and swimming count, and you can build up to more strenuous exercises as you start to feel fitter. The key is to make exercise a part of your daily routine – you'll soon find yourself running up the stairs!

WARMING UP AND COOLING DOWN

Warm-up activities are important because they ensure that your body is ready for exercise: they ease your muscles into action so that they react more readily to activity, and they also prepare you for a rise in heart rate and body temperature. Warm-ups should be done slowly and rhythmically for 5–10 minutes (depending on your age and personal fitness).

In addition, it is very important to set time aside to cool down after exercising: keep walking or moving around slowly for at least 5 minutes. This cool-down period is vital because it allows you to decrease the amount of exercise gradually. This will avoid any feelings of faintness that may be caused by the pooling of blood below the waist that occurs in the course of vigorous exercise.

MONITORING YOUR PULSE RATE

Checking your pulse rate at regular intervals is crucial because it allows you to monitor whether you are exercising adequately. The maximum heart rate for an adult is about 220 beats per minute minus your age in years. The ideal heart rate during exercise is between 65 and 80 per cent of this figure. The aim of exercise is to get your heart rate into a

WHY BOTHER WITH KEEPING FIT?

Why are you reading this book? Are you fed up with lacking confidence? Are you tired of running out of puff, being out of shape or always feeling under the weather? Do you regularly suffer from colds, or experience bad pre-menstrual syndrome (PMS), stress or sleepless nights? These are just some of the signs of being unfit. So exercise is worth it, because when you are fitter, recurring problems such as these may ease or even completely disappear.

GOLDEN RULES OF EXERCISE

- Do wear comfortable clothes and a good sports bra.
- Do invest in proper aerobic training shoes. Don't do aerobic exercise or use weights in bare feet.
- Do have a light snack, such as a small banana or a glass of fruit juice, before exercising in the evening if you haven't eaten since lunch. Don't exercise for at least an hour after a meal.
- Do take notice of injuries – don't exercise if you feel any twinges of pain.
- Do take things at your own pace and don't overtrain.
- Do drink water when exercising.

ASSESSING YOUR BODY

Everyone has features particular to their genetic make-up, but there are some general categories that people fall into. In order to be able to gain a picture of your body type and overall health you can use the evaluation methods, such as the BMI calculation and waist-to-hip ratio, outlined here.

Obviously there are certain things about your body shape, such as your height, the width of your hips and shoulders and the length of your legs, that you will never be able to change. However, it is important to focus on your good points and remember that there is much you can do to improve your natural shape.

CONFRONT YOUR BODY
Go on, be brave. Strip to your underwear, stand in front of a mirror and have a good look at your body. Take your time and be tough but realistic. You may have disliked your thighs since you were 16 – and they will probably never be those of a supermodel – but if you look hard enough you might just find that they are not as bad as you have always thought, and that improving them is not going to be that hard after all.

Note down all the areas that annoy you (and that you can do something about) as well as those that you like or

do not mind. Then go through your list of dislikes, ticking the things that you really want to do something about. Also, make a mental note to start appreciating your good points: the more you focus on them the less you will notice or mind the not-so-good zones.

Add a set of action points under the problem zones you have listed. If you want to firm up your arms to wear a sleeveless sundress, make notes like this:
• Flabby Upper Arms
• Do Basic Exercises
• Check Diet
• Exfoliate/moisturize.

Finally, add your goal(s) and your deadline to the top of the list and put it somewhere where you are going to see it frequently, such as on the refrigerator.

BODY TYPES
Although we come in a variety of shapes and sizes, the human body is cast from three basic moulds. Often, features from

Left A good way to assess your figure is to stand in front of a mirror. Be honest and look for areas that need improving.
Below Making an action checklist will help you focus on your goals and plan your campaign of action.

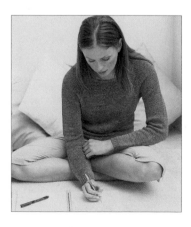

two or three of these body types are jumbled with our individual characteristics, but it is the more dominant features that slot us into one of the following groups: ectomorphs, mesomorphs and endomorphs.
Ectomorphs are usually small- and slender-framed with long limbs and narrow shoulders, hips and joints. They are thin in appearance and struggle to gain weight. Their low level of body fat makes them more susceptible to health problems. However, they are the best body type for endurance activities such as long-distance running or cycling.
Mesomorphs have medium to large – but compact – frames with broader shoulders and pelvic girdle, and well-developed muscles. The most athletic of the three body types, mesomorphs find it easy to compete in most sports and are able to build lean muscle, lose and gain weight fast, and maintain low body fat. Mesomorphs are at less risk of health problems than any other body type.
Endomorphs are naturally curvaceous, with more body fat than muscle, wider hips, shorter limbs and a lower centre of gravity than the other two body types. They are pear-shaped and often overweight. Endomorphs are likely to have the most sedentary lifestyles, have a high Body Mass Index (BMI) and are at a greater risk of poor health than any other body type.

ALTERING YOUR BODY SHAPE
You may be overweight now but this doesn't mean you have to stay that way. The right exercise and food will change your body shape and decrease the risk of health problems. Expect changes to your body shape to take time; the 21-day approach is just the beginning of your journey to a whole new you. Don't be discouraged by this. Keep the end goal in

MEASURING YOUR BMI

Use the following to find your BMI:

Metric

BMI = body mass in kilograms/divided by height x height in meters

Example:

A 1.78m tall person, weighing 79.83kg would have a BMI of 25:

79.83kg/(1.78 x 1.78)

= 79.83/3.16

= 25

Imperial

BMI = body mass in pounds/divided by height x height in inches multiplied by 703

Example:

A 5ft 10in (70in) tall person, weighing 176lb would have a BMI of 25:

176lb/(70 x 70) x 703

= 176/4,900 x 703

= 25

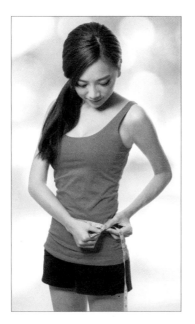

Above Measuring your waist-to-hip ratio is a very simple way of gauging your risk of health problems, and can be done at home.

ight and stay motivated. If your body hape changes too quickly, you will not ▪e able to sustain the transformation.)nce you have changed the way you ook, you will need to continue working ▪ard to maintain your new body shape.

▪ODY MASS INDEX (BMI)

▪his is a measure of a person's weight caled according to their height (see ▪ox 'Measuring Your BMI'). This is a ▪seful tool for monitoring your ▪rogress in terms of health and fitness. ▪owever, it is not accurate in all cases. ▪or example, power athletes may have ▪he same BMI score as an overweight ▪erson, even though they are carrying ▪o fat. This is because the BMI does not ▪ccount for the amount of lean muscle ▪arried. Likewise, many endurance ▪thletes have a BMI score indicating ▪hat they are underweight, even though ▪hey are a healthy weight.

In older people, BMI readings may ▪e of little use, as they will not take ▪nto account loss of muscle mass. ▪leither can the BMI be an accurate ▪neasure for children or breastfeeding

mothers. However, exceptions aside, the BMI provides a good basic guideline to follow for the general population and is a quick way to get an idea whether you are within a healthy range.

WAIST-TO-HIP RATIO

Other body measurements are also useful for monitoring health. Simply measuring your waist and hips, then calculating your waist-to-hip ratio, can be just as effective as the BMI measurement for highlighting health

risk factors. These have been found to increase if a man has a waist measurement of over 102cm/40in, or a woman has a waist measurement of more than 89cm/35in. A waist-to-hip ratio of more than 1 for men and 0.8 for women is highly detrimental to your health. At this point, the risk of heart disease, hypertension and type II diabetes is dramatically increased.

BLOOD PRESSURE

If your blood pressure is higher than 140/100, you should consult a doctor before you start any exercise routine. It is easy to measure blood pressure yourself with a blood pressure monitor. It is best to take the test before you have done any exercise that day, as exertion may affect the result. However, if you have already exercised, then make sure that you rest for at least 30 minutes before you take a blood pressure reading.

CHOLESTEROL

Your doctor can check your cholesterol level by doing a simple blood test. The result is reported in millimoles per litre (mmol/l) or milligrams per decilitre (mg/dl). A cholesterol level of 5mmol/l or 200mg/dl or less is desirable, 5 to 6 is borderline, and above 6 puts you at a high risk of a heart attack. In some places, more than half of heart attacks are linked with levels of over 5, meaning that it really is a good indication of how at risk you may be from serious health problems.

BMI AND HEALTH RISKS

Studies show that the BMI score is linked to health risk factors. Compare your score with those on the chart below. If your health risk is high or very high, you should consult a doctor and start taking exercise and eating sensibly immediately.

BMI score	Classification	Health risk
less than 18.5	underweight	moderate
18.5–24.9	normal	very low
25–29.9	overweight	low
30–34.9	obese class 1	moderate
35–39.9	obese class 2	high
above 40	extreme obesity	very high

TACKLING PROBLEM AREAS

Very few people are able to say honestly that they are totally happy with every aspect of their body. Most people have at least one gripe – whether it is flabby arms or chunky thighs. All these perceived 'flaws' can be improved by targeted exercise that improves the muscle tone of the affected region.

As anyone who has ever tried (and failed) to move the fat that commonly sits on strategic points such as hips, thighs, stomachs and buttocks knows, it is much easier to hide flaws with loose-fitting clothing than to tackle them. Trouble spots such as these are notoriously stubborn to shift, but it is possible to alter your outline with a combination of diet and exercise.

COMMON PROBLEMS

Any of the following issues can be discouraging, but has a solution.

Slack stomachs: Our stomachs become flabby when the abdominal muscles slacken; this usually happens through lack of exercise. Your abdomen extends from just under the bustline to the groin, and it is packed with muscles that criss-cross to form a wall to hold the abdominal contents in place – a bit like a corset. Exercise is not the only way to keep your stomach flat though: weight is also an important factor and the long-term answer is both diet and exercise.

Thunder thighs: Like bottoms and busts, thighs are a great source of discontent, whether it is because they are too flabby, muscular or skinny. You inherit the basic shape of your thighs, but that does not necessarily mean that you were born with

the excess fat that may be covering them. Thigh size and tone can certainly be altered with the right diet, correct body care and regular exercise. Sports such as cycling, skiing, tennis, running and riding (a great inner-muscle firmer) will tone your thighs, as will weight-training for specific areas of the body.

Large bottoms: There are three large muscles in our buttocks: gluteus maximus, medius and minimus. These create the shape, but not the size, of our rear ends. It is the tone of these muscles and the fatty tissue around them that gives us the bottoms we have. The good news is that buttock muscles respond well to exercise, which means that any effort you put into bottom-toning exercises will be rewarded quite quickly. Locomotive exercises – such as fast walking, running upstairs and jogging – are especially good bottom trimmers. Other exercises are given in the Better Buttocks routine on page 95.

Slack upper arms: Arms don't really change shape a great deal during our lives, unless we lose or gain a lot of weight. Muscle tone is the main problem, but, as in the case of thighs, exercise and specific weight-training will tone up and reshape flabby arms. It is very often the case that any changes in body shape that happen through exercise and diet are noticeable most quickly on your upper arms.

Droopy breasts: Breast shape and size only really change when our weight swings dramatically, during pregnancy, breast-feeding, menstruation, or if taking oral contraceptives. Gravity is the bust's worst enemy, especially if the breasts are not given proper support, because it literally

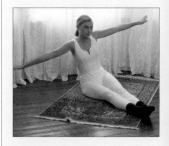
drags the breasts down and slackens their tone. Although the breasts are supported by suspensory ligaments, they do not contain any muscle (the milk glands are buffered by protective fatty tissue) so you cannot noticeably reverse lost tone. However, exercising the pectoral muscles beneath your armpits will give your breasts a firmer base and more uplift.

Thick ankles: Trim and slender ankles are seen to be a great asset. But if you are not blessed with these, or if your ankles tend

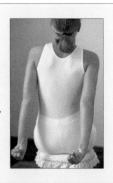

become stiff and puffy from fluid retention, you need to brush up on some ankle-improving exercises.

Assess the flexibility of your ankles by sitting on a chair with your feet on the floor and, while keeping your heel down, pull the rest of your foot up as far as it will go: if the distance between your foot and the floor measures 12–15cm/5–6in your joint flexibility is good; if it is between 10–12cm/4–5in it is fair; and if it is less than that, your joint flexibility is poor.

GOOD POSTURE

The difference that good posture makes to the look of our bodies is enormous, mainly because when we are standing properly our abdominal muscles are in their correct supporting role and the whole body is aligned so that it looks leaner and taller – meaning this is an easy way to alter your body type in

seconds! Good posture is also beneficial for our mental and physical health; some alternative therapies (such as the Alexander Technique) are based on the principle of correct posture because it can be a very effective method of easing back pain, stress and even headaches.

Strong abdominals are essential for good posture. For exercises to strengthen the abdominal muscles, see Waist Workshop on page 100 and Toned Stomach on page 101, as these focus on the core. Swimming strengthens the abs and back, too, as well as burning off fat. Check out Water Workout on page 85 for exercises you can do in the pool.

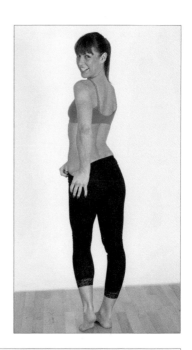

Right We all have things about our bodies we would like to change. Standing up straight and feeling confident about how we look is vital for a positive self-image.

EXERCISES TO IMPROVE YOUR POSTURE

A poor posture profile, such as a curved back, slumped shoulders and a head that juts forwards, is commonplace. Stretching exercises can help reverse this trend before the poor posture becomes habitual. Try to fit them in every day if you can, or even better, first thing in the morning and before bed.

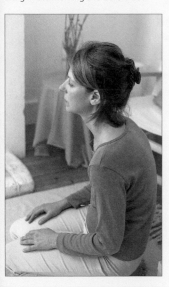

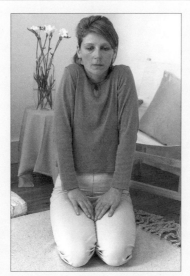

1 Take a deep breath in and slowly begin to lift your shoulders up and back as far as they will comfortably go. On the out breath, slowly release, beginning the upwards movement again on the next breath. As your shoulder blades come down, imagine them meeting in the middle of your back. Shoulder shrugs help to release tension in the large muscles of the upper back that pull on the neck.

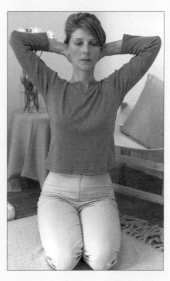

2 Centre your head and tuck in your chin. Put your hands behind your head, push your head against them and hold for 3–5 seconds. Repeat 10–20 times. Place one hand on the side of your head. With your chin in, push your head against your hand and hold for 3–5 seconds. Repeat 10–20 times. Repeat on the other side. These help to strengthen the neck muscles, which will improve your posture.

AEROBIC EXERCISES
START-UP MOVES

These exercises are an excellent way to start developing a stamina-building routine. Try to spend a couple of minutes doing each of the moves. Increase the intensity of the exercises by adding larger swinging or punching arm movements or by making the leg movements bigger or faster.

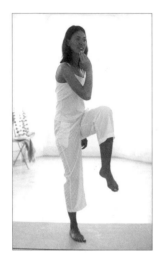

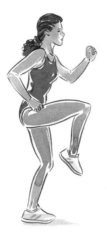

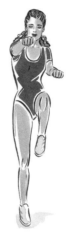

1 March in place, building up speed gradually. Lift your knees up high and swing alternate arms, as if you were running on the spot, to give yourself a full body workout.

2 Jog on the spot while 'punching' alternate arms straight out in front of you.

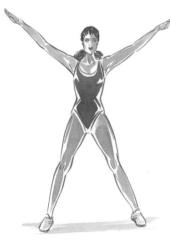

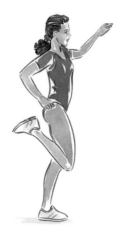

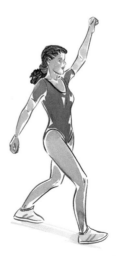

3 Do star jumps (jumping jacks) for 2 minutes. Stand with legs together and arms down by your sides. Jump so that your legs are apart, your arms are above your head and your body forms an 'X' shape. Jump back, bringing your legs together and your arms back to your sides. Repeat this movement rhythmically.

4 Bring your right heel up to your right buttock, then the left heel up to the left buttock. Keep alternating this heel-to-buttock movement as quickly as you can.

5 Move your legs forwards alternately, touching the heel to the floor. Swing or circle the arms.

START-UP STRETCHES

y this easy routine any time during the day when you have an energy dip – it's a great way to nergize yourself if you wake up tired. These are also ideal stretches to do after Start-up Moves efore you begin aerobic or stretch and tone exercises, since they work most of the muscles in the ody. The Rag Doll is especially effective since it focuses on loosening up your lower back.

HE RAG DOLL

Stand with your feet shoulder-width apart, bend your knees ightly, and let your upper body hang limply down towards the oor. Feel your back lengthen.

Breathe in and slowly curl your upper body up, keeping your nees bent and using your thigh muscles (not your back) to lift ourself. As you rise to hip level, cross your arms and continue owly curling upwards.

When your arms reach shoulder level, uncross them. Breathe ut forcefully as you extend your arms upwards. Repeat the xercise three to five times, inhaling deeply before you start ach repetition, so you create a continuous, invigorating motion.

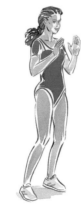

EACH TO THE CEILING

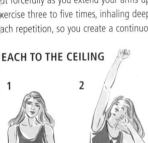

1   2

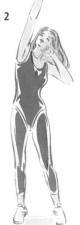

HIP ROTATION

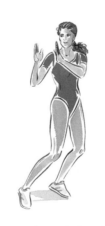

TOP TIPS

■ If possible, don't leave your workout until too late in the day, since the adrenalin coursing round your body may make it difficult for you to sleep. You may also be too tired to work out effectively, although if you have had a stressful day the exercise can help you to work off any frustration, If your do exercise late in the evening, allow enough time to finish with Essential Relaxation (page 108).

■ Eating the right foods regularly will help boost your energy levels, too. A slump after a large lunch is almost inevitable, so eat little and often. Try to consume a banana or other energy-boosting food at least an hour before exercising in the evening, so that you are able to perform well.

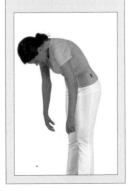

This stretching exercise relieves stress and tretches the area around the ribs, spine, and tomach muscles. Stand with your feet apart, nees slightly bent. Check your shoulders are elaxed. Breathe in slowly.

 Breathe out slowly while you reach up with our right arm, palm pointing towards the eiling. Stretch through the wrist so your hand lexes. Hold for 10 seconds as you breathe in, xhale, and stretch the left arm up as you lower he right. Repeat three times on each side.

1 Stand with feet a little more than shoulder-width apart, bend your knees, and move your arms in front of your chest with elbows bent as if you are holding a ball. Inhale deeply, relaxing your neck and shoulders, and imagine your breath filling your torso down to the base of your spine.

2 Breathe out slowly, and gently rotate your hips in a clockwise direction, stretching your hips as far as you can. Move your arms around in front in time with your hips. Repeat the movement in a counter-clockwise direction. Make 10–12 circles in alternate directions, taking your time.

BURN FAT FASTER

To lose fat from your body, you need to increase your heart rate and work hard enough to get out of breath. Try doing this fat-burning routine for 10 minutes, then follow it with other aerobic exercises, such as Dance Moves and Skipping Fit, to make up a full 30 minutes of fat-burning exercise. March in place for 2 minutes to warm up, lifting your knees high.

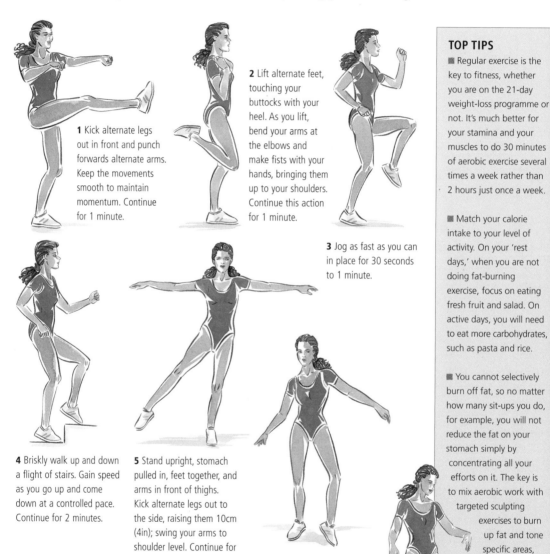

1 Kick alternate legs out in front and punch forwards alternate arms. Keep the movements smooth to maintain momentum. Continue for 1 minute.

2 Lift alternate feet, touching your buttocks with your heel. As you lift, bend your arms at the elbows and make fists with your hands, bringing them up to your shoulders. Continue this action for 1 minute.

3 Jog as fast as you can in place for 30 seconds to 1 minute.

4 Briskly walk up and down a flight of stairs. Gain speed as you go up and come down at a controlled pace. Continue for 2 minutes.

5 Stand upright, stomach pulled in, feet together, and arms in front of thighs. Kick alternate legs out to the side, raising them 10cm (4in); swing your arms to shoulder level. Continue for 2 minutes.

6 Step to the right. Bring your left foot in and tap it against the right. Step to the left and tap the right foot against the left. Take 2–4 steps in one direction before going back the other way. Continue for 1 minute.

7 Cool down for a couple of minutes by walking in place and gently shaking out your arms and legs.

TOP TIPS

■ Regular exercise is the key to fitness, whether you are on the 21-day weight-loss programme or not. It's much better for your stamina and your muscles to do 30 minutes of aerobic exercise several times a week rather than 2 hours just once a week.

■ Match your calorie intake to your level of activity. On your 'rest days,' when you are not doing fat-burning exercise, focus on eating fresh fruit and salad. On active days, you will need to eat more carbohydrates, such as pasta and rice.

■ You cannot selectively burn off fat, so no matter how many sit-ups you do, for example, you will not reduce the fat on your stomach simply by concentrating all your efforts on it. The key is to mix aerobic work with targeted sculpting exercises to burn up fat and tone specific areas, along with dieting.

DANCE MOVES

Dance-style steps are perfect to get you moving, increase your heart rate, and get your lungs working. Create your own 10-minute workout by putting on your favourite music and making up a routine from the steps shown here, plus any of the steps shown opposite, alternating them with jogging or marching in place. Start gently to give your muscles a chance to warm up.

THE GRAPEVINE

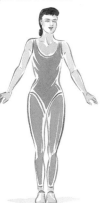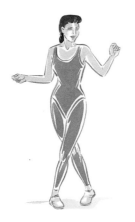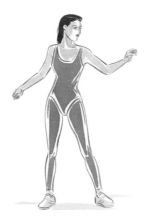

1 The grapevine is a simple step to start with. It's used as a basic element of most aerobic class routines. Stand with your feet together. Step to the left side, leading with your left foot.

2 Your right foot follows, stepping behind your left foot, so that your feet are crossed. You can work harder by using your arms during the movement. Swing them out to the side as you cross your feet and bring them in as you step again.

3 Step left again with your left leg, follow with your right foot and you step together. Keep thinking: 'Step wide, cross behind, step wide, step together.' Repeat the grapevine steps (1–3) to the right. Practice makes perfect!

THE MAMBO

This is a Latin-style step. With your feet together, step forwards diagonally with your right leg crossing your left. Allow your right hip to sway forwards, Latin-style, transfering your weight on to your front foot. Step your right foot back, allowing your hip to sway back, and bring your feet together. Repeat on the other side.

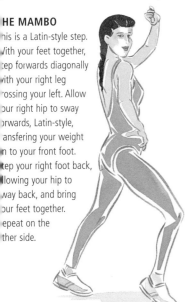

THE TURN

This move is called the pivot turn. With feet together, keep your right foot on the spot and step your left foot forwards and around, turning your body to the right, pivoting on the ball of your right foot. Take three steps to turn around until you are facing forwards again.

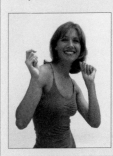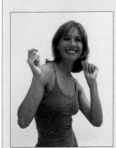

POWER-WALKING

Power-walking is a fancy name for walking briskly – roughly 1.5km (1 mile) in 12 minutes. By moving at this pace, you exercise all the major muscle groups without the high-impact action of jogging or running. Power-walk anywhere and at any time for just 10 minutes to get your heart beating, help you burn fat, and improve general fitness. It is a great activity for a lunch break!

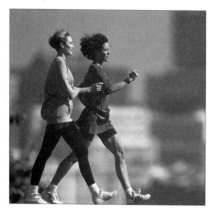

BEFORE YOU SET OUT

• To avoid dehydration, drink plenty of water before, during and after your walk. Carry water with you in a plastic bottle.

• Do the Start-up Moves (page 76) or Start-up Stretches (page 77) before you begin to power-walk. Cool down and stretch out after your walk. You will be perspiring a little and your heart rate should be raised if you have walked fast enough.

• Plan your route so that it includes some hills and is far away from major roads, if possible. Tell someone where you are going and how long you will be.

HOW TO POWER-WALK

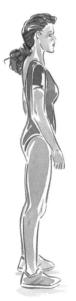
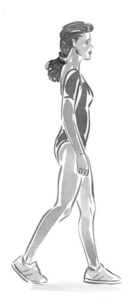
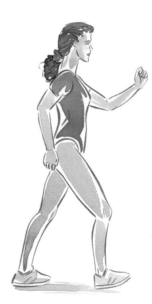

1 Before you start moving, lift your chest so that your back is straight but not arched. Relax your shoulders, keep your head high and your chin up to help you breathe efficiently and walk tall.

2 Pull your stomach in and lead from the chest. Take comfortable strides, but aim to increase their frequency – it is the speed of the walk, not the length of stride that helps to define leg muscles. Strike the ground with your heel first, then roll through to your toe.

3 Bend your arms at the elbow to form a 90-degree angle and let them swing as naturally as possible. Don't concentrate too hard on pumping your arms as this will slow you down. Focus on what you're doing – feel your leg and buttock muscles contract, and your weight shift on to your heels.

TOP TIPS

■ Avoid power-walking in areas of heavy congestion, especially if the air quality is poor. If you live in an area where the pollution levels are high, take an early morning walk when the air is at its cleanest.

■ Wear bright clothing and keep to well-lit, populated areas when out walking on your own. In rural areas, go with a friend to help you feel more secure.

■ Wear a watch – preferably one with a stop-watch facility – so you can keep a check on your times, and write them down. This will help you monitor your progress, too, which is great for motivation.

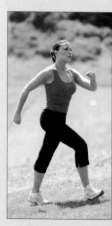

SKIPPING FIT

Skipping builds energy levels and burns off fat quickly – 10 calories a minute – the same as running. Try to avoid skipping outdoors and on concrete; it is far better to do it on a carpeted floor inside or on grass outside. You will need shoes designed for high-impact exercise and a good-quality skipping (jump) rope. The rope should be long enough to clear your head when you skip.

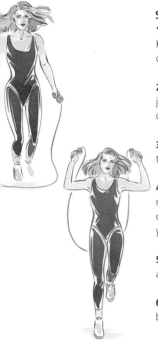

SKIP FOR STAMINA

1 Skip continuously for 1 minute, hopping with alternate feet. Keep up a slow, comfortable pace. You need plenty of space so check that you are not going to hit anything before you start.

2 Skip for 1 minute, keeping feet together. Take an extra bouncing jump in between skips if you can. This requires concentration and co-ordination, but with practice becomes easier.

3 Skip at jogging pace with alternate feet for about 2 minutes, then take up to 1 minute's rest if necessary, or keep skipping.

4 Do two 1-minute bursts at running speed, taking a 30-second rest in between. Use alternate feet rather than both feet together, or you may fall over. Shorten the jump rope by wrapping it around your hands for a harder workout if you are feeling confident.

5 Do 2 minutes' skipping at a slower, jogging pace, hopping with alternate feet.

6 Cool down with a leisurely 1-minute skip. Skipping is difficult, but with practice you will find that your technique improves.

TOP TIP

■ Skipping is high-intensity exercise and gets your heart pumping very quickly. If you can't manage 1 minute of continuous skipping to begin with, try doing 30 seconds and build up.

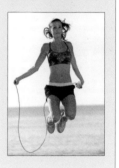

RUNNING

There is no doubt that running is one of the best ways to burn off calories fast, as well as strengthen and tone muscles and improve aerobic fitness. Just 10 minutes of running burns off around 100kcal, more if you go faster. Most people are capable of running short distances at a slow speed and, if you run regularly, you'll soon notice a big improvement in your fitness levels and your figure.

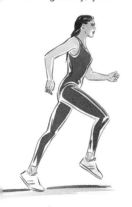

The treadmill is a good way to begin running, as the base of the machine provides some cushioning to help avoid injury. Running on a treadmill also allows you to assess your fitness as you can cover the exact distance and not be affected by terrain or weather conditions. However, treadmills don't really replicate running outside, so try both, especially if you want to carry on after the diet has finished. When running outdoors, the fresh air can cool you down and the surroundings take your mind off the exertion. Using off-road tracks will soften the impact of your foot striking the ground and will prevent injury. Try not to run on ground that is too soft, or you could slip and it will make the back of the calves work too hard and may cause injury.

Before you run, it is important that you have a warm-up, which should include at least 2 minutes of walking, 5 minutes of light jogging or fast walking, and some targeted stretches. You could walk/jog to the gym or the place where you are going to run. The best stretches will be a hamstring, quadriceps and calf stretch – the leg stretches in the Cooling Down routine on page 86 are ideal. ▶

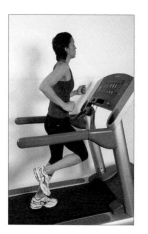

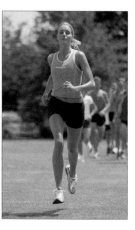

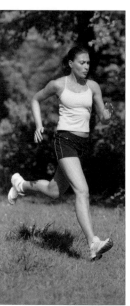

RUNNING PROGRAMME – BEGINNER

1 If you are completely new to running, begin by jogging for 1 minute and walking quickly for 2 minutes after your warm-up. Repeat this until you have been exercising for 30–45 minutes.

2 When you have completed three sessions of this combination in a week, build your jog time up to 2 minutes and walk for 1 minute for three sessions per week. Each week, add 2 minutes to your jog time.

3 If you continue in this way after the 21-day diet period has finished, after six weeks of jogging/walking three times per week, you should be able to jog for 10 minutes and walk for 1 minute for a total of 30–60 minutes.

4 Now move on to a programme for a more experienced runner, outlined below, and build your frequency and distance. You may consider joining a running group.

RUNNING PROGRAMME – EXPERIENCED

1 If at the start of the diet you are able to jog for 10 minutes and walk for 1 minute for a total of 30–60 minutes, try to jog continuously for 15–20 minutes.

2 Time yourself over distances of 2km/1.2 miles and 5km/3.1 miles once a week. This will allow you to measure your improvement and set new targets. To maximize the benefits and avoid injury, aim for a steady rate of improvement – your body needs

a chance to build the correct muscles and establish stability to cope with the physical demands of running.

3 You can now include some longer runs at a steady pace lasting for 30–40 minutes. It is better to run for longer at a slightly slower pace in order to burn fat and improve endurance, especially if you are aiming for distance rather than speed. You can build speed later.

BUILDING FREQUENCY AND DISTANCE AFTER THE DIET

1 Increase your training by 10 per cent a week, so if you run for 30 minutes four times a week, add 10–15 minutes the next week, then 20 minutes, and so on.

2 Running more often should be your goal before increasing mileage, as this helps to build the habit of regular running and gives your metabolism a boost every day. This may mean shortening your route temporarily, for example you might go from three half-hour sessions to five 20-minute sessions. After that, try adding 5 minutes every week until you are running 40–45 minutes, five or six times per week.

3 As well as running more often and for slightly longer each time, you should plan one long run per week, aiming to build up to between 90 minutes and 2 hours. This will teach your body to be more efficient at using fat for fuel, which means your body fat levels will drop and you will be able to run farther comfortably.

4 Think in terms of time rather than distance to begin with so that you discover your natural pace, which will help you work out how far you are running. Remember the 10 per cent rule – don't build up your long run on the same weeks that you increase your other runs.

TOP TIPS

■ Running is an impact activity that puts some strain on joints. Seek professional advice if you have injuries or joint problems, as this activity may not be for you.

■ Comfortable footwear that absorbs impact is vital; you will need running trainers that have been specifically designed to provide the proper support and cushioning. Visit a store where the sales advisors are trained to watch you and suggest shoes that suit your style. If possible, test on a treadmill before you buy them.

■ Wear comfortable, breathable clothes. If it is cold, wear tights to trap body heat. This is important to protect joints with poor blood supply, such as your knees. On your top half, wear a few layers so that you can take them off and on as required. Wear a cap to keep the sun off your head and to prevent sweat from getting into your eyes.

■ Record your mileage and make sure you replace your shoes after about 800km (500 miles).

■ Carry water to maintain your hydration.

■ Keep your pace easy, so you are able to chat or sing as you run.

MACHINE WORKOUT

If you are a member of a gym or have a access to a machine elsewhere, then make use of it to really burn off some calories. Fast walking or light bicycling both burn about 40 calories in 10 minutes. Bicycling hard uses 100 calories in 10 minutes. You can either exercise on one machine for the full 30 minutes, or swap around if you prefer, exercising for 10 minutes on each, as outlined below.

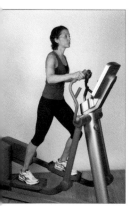

10-MINUTE CROSS-TRAINER

1 Move at a moderate to fast pace at a low resistance for 2 minutes to warm up. Move your arms in an exaggerated way so you are getting a total body workout.

2 Continue at the same moderate pace, but increase the resistance for 2 minutes so you are pushing hard to move the handles and foot pads and feel your heart rate increasing.

3 Switch the machine back to a medium resistance and increase your speed so you start to move more quickly, at a pace that will be sustainable for 5 minutes. If you really struggle, reduce the resistance setting rather than your speed.

4 Reduce your speed and the resistance so you are moving at a moderate pace to help you cool down slowly for 1 minute.

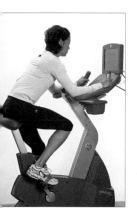

10-MINUTE CYCLE

1 Set the machine to a fairly low resistance if you are new to cycling, or make it harder if you feel fit. Cycle slowly for 1 minute to warm up your muscles.

2 Increase your speed and bicycle for up to 5 minutes at a moderately fast pace. It is better to set the machine to a medium resistance and be able to turn your legs quickly than use a hard resistance and struggle to pedal.

3 Switch the bicycle machine to uphill and pedal for another 3 minutes. Keep pushing; the end is in sight and this resistance training helps to burn off fat and improve cardiovascular and aerobic fitness.

4 Switch back to a flat gradient and reduce your speed and the resistance for the last minute, to cool down slowly. Adjust the resistance as you get fitter.

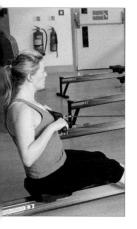
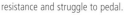

10-MINUTE ROW

1 Set a fairly low resistance on the machine. Pull the handle in towards your stomach as you glide back and forth on the seat. Do this slowly for 2 minutes.

2 Increase the speed at which you row and pull the handle in towards your stomach as you move back and forth on the seat. Keep the motion smooth and strong, not jerky and uncoordinated. Continue for 5 minutes.

3 For 1 minute only, concentrate really hard on keeping your arm movements as strong and as fast as you can. Imagine you are in a boat race and are heading towards the finish line.

4 Gradually slow down your rowing speed for 2 minutes, but try not to lose momentum. Continue to keep your arm movements strong and smooth as you cool down slowly. As you improve, increase the resistance.

TOP TIPS

■ If you are fit and want to focus on just one machine, these 10-minute workouts can be adapted to last for 30 minutes. Follow the same warm-up, then simply extend the amount of time spent cross-training, cycling or rowing at a steady speed on a medium resistance, so that the workout lasts longer. You may need to go more slowly than you would for a 10-minute session. Cool down in the same way.

■ When buying or borrowing an exercise machine for home use or when using one in the gym, make sure you understand how it works. Get an expert to show you all the features and the correct techniques for using it. Injury can occur if your technique is bad or you don't understand how to change the speed or stop.

■ When buying machines, go to a reputable store and test all the models. It is probably better to go for something that is mid-range in terms of price – if it's too cheap, the machine can be flimsy.

PUTTING UP A FIGHT

Boxing moves improve coordination, build up stamina, make your body stronger, and help you get rid of pent-up aggression. Many boxers skip as a warm-up, so you could lead up to this routine by doing the Start-up Moves (page 76), then 10 minutes of Skipping Fit (page 81) and finish with the Burn Fat Faster routine (page 78). You will need a wooden pole or broom handle for the lifting lunge

SIDE KICKS

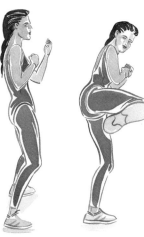

1 Stand with your knees slightly bent, hands held in fists, elbows bent, and hands up in front of your body at shoulder height.

2 Tilt your right hip forwards and kick your right leg out to the side, leading with your buttock muscle. Keep your foot flexed. Repeat 15 times. Switch legs.

LIFTING LUNGE

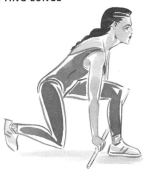

1 Lunge your right leg out in front, foot flat on the floor, making a 90-degree angle with your knee. The knee should not go beyond your ankle. Keep the left leg behind, directly under the hip. Slide a stick or broom handle under your right knee. Your back should be straight and your stomach held in tight.

PUNCHING

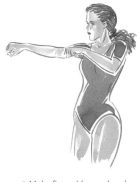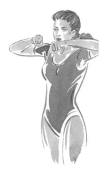

1 Make fists with your hands, backs of hands facing the ceiling, and punch your arms straight out in front of you. Continue for 2 minutes and then relax.

2 Draw your fists up close to your face and make short punching movements in the air. Increase your speed. After 2 minutes repeat step 1.

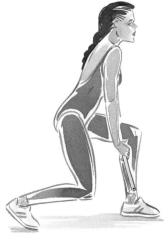

2 Lift and lower the broom handle slowly from under your right knee to the floor 10 times – your left knee should try to touch the floor and you will feel the muscles working. Change legs and repeat for another 10 repetitions. This exercise works the arms, thighs, and buttocks.

TOP TIPS

■ If you enjoy doing these boxing moves, you can learn more by watching a boxercise DVD or attending a class, where you can use a punchbag to get rid of pent-up aggression!

■ Skipping makes an excellent warm-up for boxing exercises and is a good aerobic activity, which is why so many professional boxers do it. You can extend this routine by Skipping Fit (page 81) after your warm-up stretches and before you go into the boxing exercises.

■ Remember to drink plenty of water before, during, and after strenuous exercise. Put a bottle of water out ready before you begin an exercise routine so that it is within easy reach.

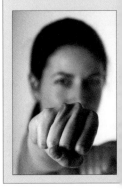

WATER WORKOUT

Exercising in water builds stamina, strength and flexibility, and there is no danger of straining joints because the water bears your weight. The pressure of the water also provides resistance and makes your muscles work harder. Use this 10-minute underwater exercise sequence as a warm-up prior to swimming laps for 20 minutes. Doing fast breast-stroke for 10 minutes burns off about 90 calories.

WALKING THROUGH WATER

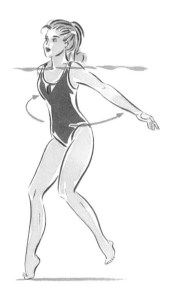

In water up to your shoulders, walk as fast as you can, pushing your arms forwards and around in large sweeping movements under water. This is excellent for burning off fat and providing good all-over conditioning. Your legs get a good workout because they have to work against the force of the water; your stomach muscles are used more than if you were walking on land; and the upper back muscles and the pectoral muscles also get exercised. Continue for 2 minutes, or for longer if possible.

LEG LIFTS

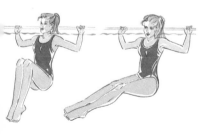

With your back pressed against the side of the pool, hold on to the edge as you lift and lower your legs, keeping them bent at the knees. Continue in this way for 2–3 minutes. This will work the muscles at the front of the hip as well as the buttock muscles. Bend, then straighten your legs out in front of you without lowering them to work the fronts and backs of your thighs. Continue for 2–3 minutes.

RUN IN DEEP WATER

Make running or cycling movements underwater using your hands to keep afloat. If you are not a confident swimmer, you might feel more comfortable wearing a light life jacket to keep you afloat. Try to run from one side of the pool to the other. This works all the muscles in your legs and arms, and keeps your heart and lungs in good working order. It also quickly burns up calories. Try doing this for 2 minutes and build up to more as your stamina increases.

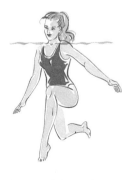

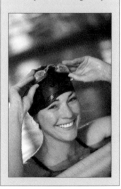

COOLING DOWN

Take time to stretch your muscles after all strenuous aerobic exercise. This will protect you from cramps and help reduce muscle stiffness. Stretching work done while your muscles are warm has the double benefit of cooling you down and helping you to keep flexible. You can also use these stretches at the end of a busy day to de-stress yourself.

FLEXIBILITY STRETCH

1 Lie flat on your back with your stomach pulled in and your lower back pressed into the floor. Bend your right leg, keeping your right foot on the floor. Raise your left leg, sole towards the ceiling.

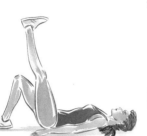

2 Clasp your left leg with both hands around the thigh or calf and gently pull your leg towards you. Stop when you feel the stretch, and before feeling any strain. Hold for 10–20 seconds, then relax and repeat both steps on the right leg.

LEG STRETCHES

SHAKE OUT

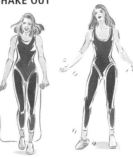

1 If you have been doing intense aerobic exercise, slow down gradually, keeping going at a leisurely pace for a few minutes before coming to a complete stop.

2 Shake your arms and legs out to help prevent stiffness and help you cool down.

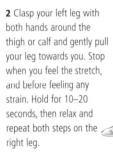

2 Take a big stride forwards with your left foot. Check your hips are facing forwards and feet are flat on the floor. The left leg should be slightly bent. Hold the stretch for a count of 20. Repeat on the right leg.

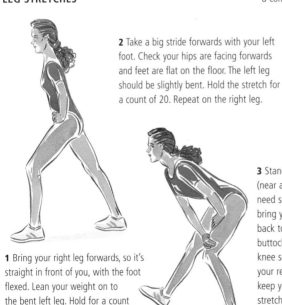

1 Bring your right leg forwards, so it's straight in front of you, with the foot flexed. Lean your weight on to the bent left leg. Hold for a count of 10, release, and repeat on the other side.

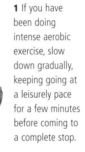

3 Stand upright (near a wall if you need support) and bring your left heel back towards your left buttock. Bend your right knee slightly, tuck your rear under, and keep your knees together. Feel the stretch in the front of your thighs. Hold for 10–20 seconds, relax, and release. Repeat on the right leg.

TOP TIPS

■ Don't suddenly stop if you get tired during aerobic exercise. This could make you feel faint. When you exercise, your heart rate increases and your muscles produce a pumping action to accommodate the increased blood flow and speed the return of blood to the heart. If you stop suddenly, this pumping action also stops and the rate of blood flow into the muscles remains fast. The result is a pooling of blood in the veins that can make you feel light-headed and dizzy. Even if you feel tired, try to continue the exercise at a slow speed for a couple of minutes or walk to cool down.

■ If you cramp as you are cooling down, slowly walk around until the spasm subsides, stretch out and have a drink.

■ If you have time, finish your cool down by relaxing for 10 minutes, following the Essential Relaxation routine on page 108. This is especially beneficial if you exercise in the evening, as it will help you sleep.

MOVING ON

Once you have got used to exercising during the 21-day weight-loss plan, you will find that you want to – and can – do more. To continue improving your fitness, you will need to carry on doing between three and five aerobic sessions per week, with each session lasting at least 30 minutes. You may want to join a class or gym, but there are lots of other fun ways to exercise too.

Walk more
Increase the pace and distance you walk. Setting a brisk pace while you walk can burn off 150 calories in 30 minutes. If you live near, or are on holiday near, a beach, walk in the sand barefoot. It's harder work, so exercises you more, and is especially good for toning your calves, but don't overdo it.

Try jogging farther
If you have followed the running programme for beginners on page 82, you should be able to start to run for longer by the time you finish the 21-day programme. If you can already run for 30 minutes, try increasing the distance and frequency and aim to speed up or incorporate some hills.

Head for the hills
Get out into the country and try hill walking. This shapes your legs, particularly your thighs and calves, as well as your buttocks. It also burns more calories than walking on the flat. Do not slump forwards when you go uphill – carry your neck and spine straight, keep your shoulders pulled back and stomach tucked in. Control your strides going downhill and keep the same upright posture.

4 Swim yourself fitter
Go swimming more often to build stamina and endurance. Water is weight-bearing, so swimming is safe for pregnant women, the unfit, those with back or joint problems, and the elderly. Warm up by doing the Water Workout on page 85, then swim laps continuously for maximum benefit. Aim for 30 minutes and build up to 60 minutes.

5 Enjoy a sport
Play a social sport, such as tennis, badminton, or squash. Most of these sports are played for 30–60 minutes. Try to play with people of the same experience and fitness level as you, so you don't push yourself too hard or lose motivation.

6 Work and play
Mix and match exercise routines and chores to fit 30 minutes of continuous activity into a busy schedule. For example, do 20 minutes' gardening, followed by 10 minutes' skipping.

7 Get a full body workout
Combine aerobic exercise with stretching and toning for a full body workout. Aim to follow your 30 minutes of aerobic exercise

with at least 10 minutes of toning, and include two 30-minute (or more) sessions of just toning on your 'rest' days.

8 Mow the lawn and build stamina
Gardening is good for you – 10 minutes' weeding burns 35 calories. Mowing the lawn burns up to 50 calories in 20 minutes. Mowing uphill burns another 25 calories, builds stamina and provides a resistance weight for toning up your arms.

9 Snack and stay slim
One hour's hard housework burns off 250kcal – the same as bicycling for 30 minutes. When you have finished, reward yourself with a tasty, healthy snack if you feel hungry. Resist the temptation to sit down with a cookie or doughnut!

10 Dust and stretch
Dusting burns up 25 calories in 10 minutes, but you can adapt it to work in some stretches plus arm toning and strengthening. Use a feather duster to skim around the ceiling corners. Stretch your arm high and bend slightly to one side. Hold for 10–20 seconds. Then work the other side of your body.

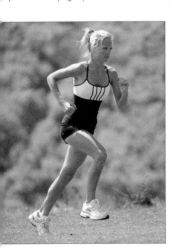
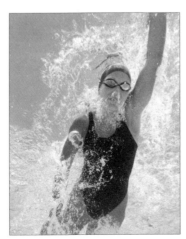
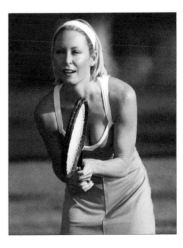

STRETCH AND TONE
TOTAL-BODY WARM-UP

This simple routine should be done before the start of any toning and stretching exercise routine to help warm up and stretch the muscles, so preventing the risk of injury.

GET READY, GET SET, GO!

1 First warm up the lower back. Bend forwards about 30 degrees, placing your hands above your kneecaps to support your back. Round out and then straighten your spine eight times.

2 Stand tall and march in place for 1 minute. Increase the pace for 1 minute, lifting your legs higher. Step from side to side, bringing one foot in to tap against the other, for 1 minute. Jog gently in place for 1 minute.

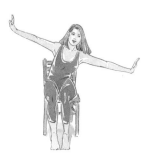

3 Stand with your feet apart or sit. Stretch your arms out and bend to the left to stretch your side. Hold for a count of eight, then repeat on the right side.

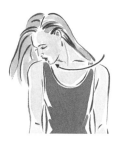

4 Gently drop your head on to your chest and slowly circle it to the left towards your left shoulder. Circle back to the centre, then to the right. Repeat five times.

5 Shrug your shoulders up towards your ears. Slowly rotate your shoulders forwards, then back to the centre and backwards. Keep repeating this motion for 30 seconds.

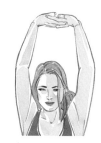

6 Stand and stretch your arms up so that they are either side of your ears. Link your fingertips and turn your palms towards the ceiling. Stretch and hold for a count of eight. Relax and repeat.

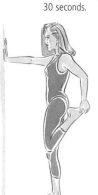

7 Stand in front of a wall or chair and press one hand on to the wall or hold on for support. Keeping your right knee soft, bend your left leg, tucking your heel into your buttock. Clasp your foot with your left hand and hold for 10. Feel the stretch in your front thigh. Change legs and repeat.

8 Stand with your legs wide apart, toes turned out and feet flat on the floor. Make your hands into fists in front of your thighs. With your stomach and buttocks tucked in, slowly bend your knees, keeping your heels on the floor, curling your arms up to your shoulders. Relax back into the starting position and repeat the movement for up to 1 minute.

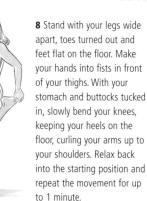

TOP TIPS

■ Frequency, not intensity, is the key to stretching effectively and improving flexibility. Ideally, try to do these warm-up exercises every morning when you wake up, even if you do not do any other exercise.

■ To avoid post-exercise aches and pains, you must stretch out after you exercise, too, whether you have been doing stamina-building or toning exercises. See Cooling Down on page 86 and Stretch It Out on page 105.

■ Gentle daily exercise can help to prevent minor aches and pains and also help you to combat stress.

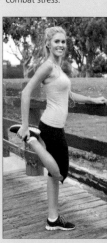

EFFORTLESS EXERCISE

Start getting fit by introducing exercise into your life at every opportunity, not just during the specific time you set aside each day to exercise while on the weight-loss programme. Here are some routines you can do around the house – waiting for a kettle to boil or while watching a television programme. All you need is a chair and tin cans or bottles of water to use as weights.

UPPER ARMS

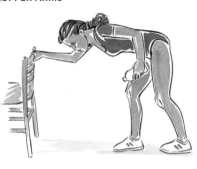

Stand an arm's length from a chair. Put your right foot in front of your left, hip-width apart. Keeping knees soft, lean forwards from your hips until your body is parallel to the floor. Put your right hand on the chair for support. Holding a weight in your left hand, bend your left elbow and hold it close to your waist. Straighten your left arm behind you. Pause and bend back to starting position. Repeat 10 times, then change sides.

WAIST

Holding weights, stand upright, feet hip-width apart, arms resting down by your sides. Keep your back and shoulders straight and slowly bend at the waist down to the right without twisting. Try to reach your right hand down towards your ankle. Feel the stretch in your waist. Raise yourself up to the starting position, then stretch over to the left. Repeat the movement slowly up to 20 times on each side – do not bounce or jerk your body as you make the movement.

TOP TIPS

■ Turn the radio to a channel playing music with a beat, and dance or just jump around energetically for 2 minutes continuously. This will boost your heart rate, stamina and circulation. It will also help warm you up for these simple stretching exercises.

■ Tone your legs while you are in the bath. Bend your left leg and stretch out your right leg in front of you. Raise and lower the right leg slowly 20 times. Swap legs and repeat the exercise.

■ Circle your wrists and ankles while lying in the bathtub. This is especially helpful to reduce swelling caused by fluid retention.

LEG STRETCHER

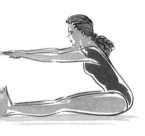

Do this simple exercise against the wall. Stretch your arms out in front of you at shoulder level. Reach slowly forwards as if someone is pulling your hands, but don't arch your back. Feel a slight stretch in the back of your legs and hold for 10 seconds. Return to the starting position and repeat the exercise up to 10 times.

LEG SHAPER

Stand, feet hip-width apart, arms by your sides (use some weights to give you extra balance if you like). Lower your buttocks as if you are going to sit on a chair. Don't squat down too low and keep your heels on the floor. Slowly return to your starting position and repeat up to 10 times.

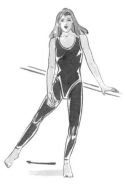

THIGH SHAPER

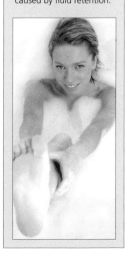

Hold a work surface or the back of a chair with your left hand. Tighten your stomach and buttock muscles. Bend your left leg and lift your right foot out to the side. Keeping your body tall, lift and lower the leg 10 times. Turn around and repeat.

WORK WORKOUT

You can tone up flabby muscles, burn fat and increase your energy levels on the way to work, sitting at your desk and again on the way home. Try these toning exercises on the bus, train or tram. If you work above the first floor, start taking the stairs instead of the elevator for a couple of flights and walk up them quickly. Your stamina and strength will soon increase if you do this twice daily.

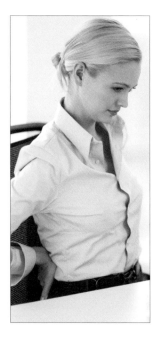

UPPER BODY STRETCH

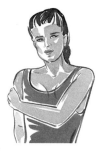

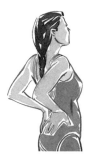

1 Sit upright in your chair, feet flat on the floor, your stomach muscles pulled in. Reach your left arm across the front of your body. Pull back your right arm to pull the left arm closer into your chest. Feel the stretch in your left arm and shoulder. Hold for 10–15 seconds. Repeat with the right arm.

2 Stand up. Pull your stomach in tight and position your hands at the top of your buttocks. Slowly push your elbows closer together, until they are nearly touching. Open up your chest to the ceiling and expand your rib cage. Hold for 10 seconds. Repeat five times. This exercise is good for relieving tension.

TOP TIPS

■ Prevent back ache, look slimmer and appear taller by improving your posture when walking or standing. You can do this anywhere – simply stand up straight with your stomach and buttocks pulled in. If you hold this posture often enough, it will soon feel natural to you and you will feel odd when you slouch. The other great benefits of improving your posture are improved all-over muscle tone, and your clothes will look better on you, too!

■ If possible, use your lunch break to go for a power-walk or swim for half an hour. This will improve your energy levels for the afternoon and will make you less likely to succumb to a mid-afternoon slump.

■ Walk briskly or bicycle all or part of the way to work – especially when the weather is good. You may find it an effort at first, but after a week or two you won't tire so easily and it is a great way to fit in your daily exercise.

UPPER BODY STRETCH

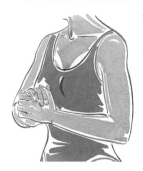

Sit with your hands, palms together, in your lap or in front of you at roughly waist height. Squeeze your palms together hard for a count of five and release. Repeat the movement up to 10 times. This is a good exercise to do when you are stuck in a traffic jam.

THIGH TONER

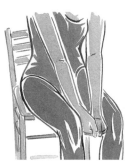

Tuck in your stomach muscles and sit tall in your chair. Make your hands into fists and place them between your knees. Alternatively, place a book bag or briefcase between your knees. Squeeze in with your thighs for a count of 50. Release and repeat as many times as you like.

BUTTOCK BUSTER

Do this exercise while you stand by the photocopier at work or while you are at the sink at home. Tighten your buttocks, hold in your stomach and, keeping your knees slightly bent and soft, move your left leg 5cm (2in) out behind you, with the foot off the floor. Hold for a count of 10, release and repeat the action on the other side. Alternate legs. Keep going for as long as possible.

UPPER BODY TONE

Flabby arms, saggy breasts and a thick waist are all common complaints, but they are relatively easy to reverse with regular toning and a healthier diet. These simple exercises will sculpt and strengthen your arms, shoulders, chest and waist and can be done anywhere there is a bench, chair, desk or bed at the right height – from the gym and living room to work or even in the bedroom.

UPPER BODY STRETCH

1 Sit on the edge of the bench, chair, bed or other surface, knees bent, toes pointing forwards, and hands shoulder-width apart beneath your buttocks, hands gripping the edge of the surface for support.

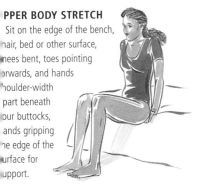

2 Bend your arms as you lower your buttocks to the floor, holding your stomach in. Just before you reach the floor raise yourself back up, pushing down with your arms as you raise your body up. Repeat 10 times.

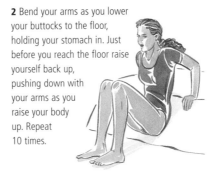

CHEST PRESS

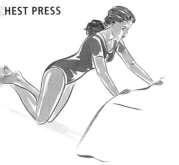

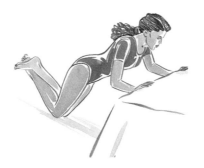

1 Kneel on the floor, on a folded towel if you need to. Position your hands on the surface slightly wider than shoulder-width apart, fingers pointing forwards and then cross your ankles.

2 Lower your chest towards the surface. Keep your stomach pulled in and your body straight from head to knees. Push away from the surface. Repeat 10 times and work up to more.

WAIST CURLS

1 Lie on the floor with the lower part of your legs resting over the edge of the surface, your back pressed firmly into the floor. Loosely position your right hand behind your head and stretch your left hand out to the side.

2 Pull in your abdominal muscles and curl up towards the surface, lifting from your waist. Twist to the left, leading with your right shoulder, not your elbow. Slowly return to starting position. Repeat 10 times. Repeat on the other side.

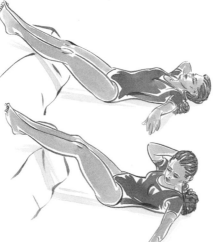

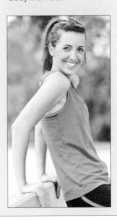

LOWER BODY TONE

You don't have to be a member of a gym to do these toning moves, so you have no excuse not to work that body. Begin by doing the Total-body Warm-up routine on page 88 to get the blood flowing and avoid injuring yourself. You will need a couple of pillows and a mat or towel to lie on for this quick but highly effective lower body workout.

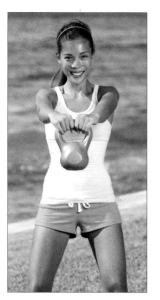

SUPER SQUATS

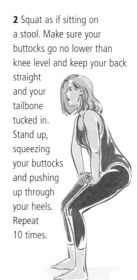

1 Stand with your arms resting on the tops of your thighs or crossed in front of you. Squat down with feet hip-width apart, toes pointing forwards, heels on the floor. Pull in your stomach, tilt your pelvis so your tailbone is tucked under and try not to arch your back.

2 Squat as if sitting on a stool. Make sure your buttocks go no lower than knee level and keep your back straight and your tailbone tucked in. Stand up, squeezing your buttocks and pushing up through your heels. Repeat 10 times.

TOP TIPS

■ Men and women store fat differently. Women tend to accumulate fat around their stomachs, hips and thighs. This is why it is important to exercise these areas as activity helps to improve shape and muscle tone and to reduce the appearance of cellulite.

■ If you are totally new to exercise, you may find it hard to complete the recommended number of repetitions. Don't worry – increase the number of repetitions over a few sessions, working to the point where the muscle being trained feels slightly tired. Do one more repetition, then stop. Listen to your body and stop if you feel tired or have any twinges.

■ Combine these exercises with the ones in Better Buttocks (p95), Inner Thigh Tone (p96) and Outer Thigh Tone (p97) for a full lower body workout.

■ To make the squats harder and really work your body, hold a weight out in front of you while you do them, as shown in the photo.

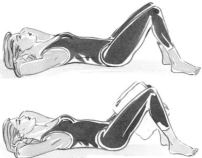

INNER THIGH SQUEEZE

1 Lie on your back on the floor with your hands behind your head. Keep your knees bent and your feet slightly apart. Do not arch your back.

2 Position a folded pillow between your knees. Breathe in and, as you breathe out, squeeze the pillow hard between your thighs. Hold your stomach in and press your lower back firmly into the floor as you do this. Hold for at least 2 seconds, release slowly, and repeat 10 times.

STREAMLINED STOMACH

1 Lie on a mat on the floor with the lower part of your legs resting on a raised surface and your back pressed firmly into the floor. Loosely position your hands behind your head. (Never pull yourself up with your hands as this can strain your neck.)

2 Pull in your stomach, then breathe out and slowly curl your body upwards so that your head and shoulders, but not your lower back, leave the floor. Lower yourself back down. Repeat 10 times and build up to more.

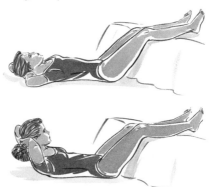

SUPER SHOULDERS

Exercising your shoulders can improve the shape of your body, making your shoulders look slightly wider, your waist look smaller and giving your upper body more of a 'triangular' shape. Most of us don't worry about our shoulders because it is not an area that accumulates fat, but it is worth trying these routines to improve your shape and flexibility. March in place for a few minutes to warm up.

SHOULDER PRESSES

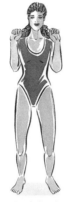
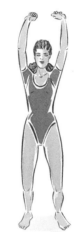

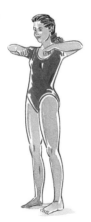
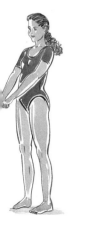

1 Stand with feet hip-width apart, knees soft, arms down to the sides, elbows bent, and hands at shoulder height. Hold in abdominals and buttocks.

2 Slowly push your arms up straight with your palms towards the ceiling. Do not lock your elbows. Slowly lower your arms. Repeat 10 times.

PULL-UPS

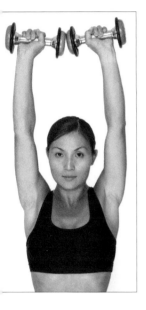

Stand with your feet hip-width apart, arms forwards, elbows at waist height. Hold in your abdominals and tighten your buttocks. Hold weights if you like.

2 Pull your elbows back and squeeze between the shoulder blades as you pull arms up to shoulder level. Return to starting position. Repeat 10 times.

PUSH-UPS

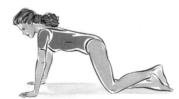

1 On a mat or towel on the floor, position yourself on your knees, feet on the floor and ankles crossed. Place your arms directly under your shoulders, hands straight out in front.

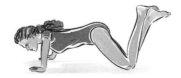

2 Using your arms, lower yourself slowly towards the floor as far as you can, pulling in your stomach and buttock muscles. Repeat 10 times. As you get stronger, keep your feet off the floor.

TOP TIPS

■ Most of us carry one shoulder higher than the other, as a result of tensing the area through stress, and doing things such as holding the telephone receiver between the jaw and shoulder, and carrying a heavy bag on one side. Learn to relax your shoulders, avoid cradling the telephone receiver against your shoulder, and when carrying things try to distribute the weight evenly.

■ To relieve tension in the shoulders, try the Work Workout exercises outlined on page 90. These simple stretches can be done at your desk or on a journey.

■ The skin on the shoulders and the back often gets neglected and may be dull-looking or suffer from spots. Exfoliate and cleanse these zones regularly to keep the skin looking good.

■ To make the shoulder presses and pull-ups harder, hold light weights in your hands. You can make your own by filling empty water bottles with sand or rice.

TRIMMER ARMS

Trim, toned upper arms are not just for the young and super-fit. The exercises here strengthen the bicep and tricep (back of arm) muscles. You can tone up these areas relatively quickly with a few simple but regular exercises. You will need a firm chair, a wall for support and weights. March in place for a few minutes or do the Total Body Warm-up (p88) before you begin.

WALL PUSH-UP

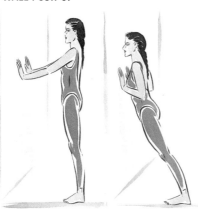

1 Stand facing a wall with your feet hip-width apart and your arms stretched out in front of you. Place your palms flat on the wall, positioning them roughly in line with your rib cage.

2 Bend your elbows and push your body weight on to your arms, aiming your nose towards the wall and keeping your hips directly under your shoulders. Push out. Repeat 10 times.

BICEP CURLS

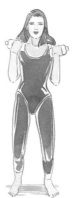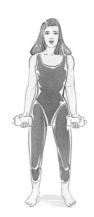

1 Stand with feet hip-width apart, knees soft. With a weight in each hand, bend your arms at the elbows. Bring up to your shoulders, keeping your elbows close to your body.

2 Lower your arms slowly to the starting position, making sure your elbows do not lock as you lower and extend your arms. Repeat the exercise 10 times.

CHAIR DIP

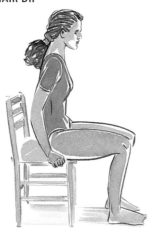

1 Sit on the edge of a firm, stable chair. Keep your feet hip-width apart and hold on to the chair with your fingers gripping the edge of the seat.

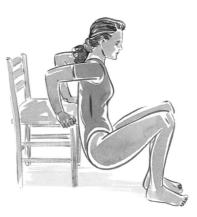

2 Lower your buttocks slowly towards the floor, using your arms to support your weight. Ease back up, feeling the stretch in the back of your arms. Repeat 10 times, and build up to more.

TOP TIPS

■ Combine bicep curls with squats for an upper and lower body workout in one. Squat down as though you are going to sit on a low stool (for an illustration of this see the Super Squats sequence on page 92). As you do so, bend your elbows and slowly bring your forearms into your chest. Return to the starting position slowly and repeat the move 10 times, building up to more as you get fitter.

■ Breathe out on the hardest part of each exercise. Breathe in as you go down in dips and curls and as you bend your elbows during push-ups; breathe out with the effort of returning to the starting position.

■ The skin around the tops of your arms, especially on the back, can get dimply due to cellulite or it may be bumpy and dull due to poor skin tone and lack of exfoliation. For ways to improve the condition of your skin, check out page 114, pages 116–17 and page 119 for top tips on exfoliating and moisturizing techniques.

BETTER BUTTOCKS

To get your buttocks into shape, try these simple but powerful exercises. Do the Total Body Warm-up routine on page 88 or march in place for a few minutes before you begin. For the leg lunges and buttock toner, work on a non-slip surface such as a gym mat. It is best to do this, and most toning and stretching exercises, with bare feet as they grip much better than socks.

BUTTOCK SHAPER

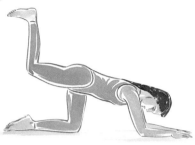 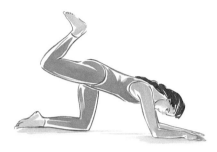

1 Put a towel or mat on the floor and position yourself on your knees, resting the upper part of your body on your elbows. Holding your stomach muscles in tightly, bend one leg up, flexing the foot. Keeping the foot flexed, lift the knee upwards towards the ceiling until you feel the buttocks contract. Lower the leg and repeat 10 times. Next, hold the raised leg position and 'pulse' the leg upwards, making small, fast movements for a count of 10.

2 Now squeeze up and move the heel inwards, about 15cm (6in), towards your buttocks. First lift the leg, curl in the heel, then release and lower slightly. Repeat 10 times. Do the entire sequence on the other leg.

Do the Total Body Warm-up routine on page 88

LEG LUNGES

1 Stand with feet hip-width apart. Turn your left foot in slightly. Step forwards about 90cm (3ft) with your right foot. Check your hips are facing forwards. Relax your shoulders, lift your chest and contract your stomach and buttocks.

2 Breathe in and lower your left thigh and bend your right knee. Make sure your right knee does not go in front of your toes and your rear end does not drop below the line of your knee. Return to the starting position and repeat 10 times, working alternate legs.

BUTTOCK TONER

1 Stand behind a firm chair or work surface with feet hip-width apart. Pull in your stomach and buttocks. Go on to tiptoes, hold for a few seconds, and lower. Repeat 10 times.

2 Stand with your feet shoulder-width apart and toes out. Go on tiptoes and bend your knees, keeping your back straight and taking your buttocks no lower than the knees. Lower heels to the floor. Repeat 10 times.

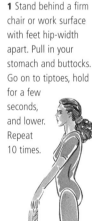

TOP TIPS

■ Take the stairs whenever you can and take them two at a time. This will give your buttocks an effective mini-workout.

■ Whenever you find yourself standing during the day (standing in line, or on the bus, for example), clench your buttocks tightly and release. Do this as often as you can, and there should be a marked improvement in muscle tone within weeks.

■ It is essential that you don't put any stress on the knees and back. Do not step so far forwards or backwards that you cannot return to standing without putting pressure on the lower back or losing your balance or posture. Do the exercises in front of a mirror occasionally so you can check your posture.

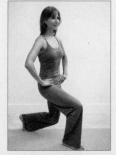

INNER THIGH TONE

Inner thighs are prone to flabbiness and most women would like to firm them up, even if they are slim. These exercises will tighten and tone up the area and improve circulation. Warm up before starting by marching in place for a few minutes or doing the Total-body Warm-up (p88). You will need a mat or towel to lie on and a firm chair for support.

INNER THIGH PRESS

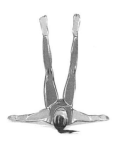

1 Lie on your back. Raise your legs slowly, keeping your knees slightly bent. Make sure your neck is relaxed and your head is on the floor.

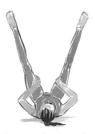

2 Place your hands on the insides of your thighs. Hold in your abdominals, pushing out with your hands while you push in with your thighs.

BASIC PLIÉ

1 Hold on to the back of a chair. Stand up straight with your feet a little wider than shoulder-width apart and your feet turned out slightly.

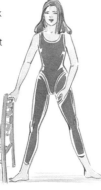

2 Keeping your heels on the floor and your buttocks tucked in, slowly bend your knees, making sure your buttocks go no lower than your knees. Repeat up to 10 times.

INNER THIGH RAISE

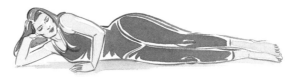

1 Lie on your right side, propped up on your right forearm. Breathe regularly and evenly.

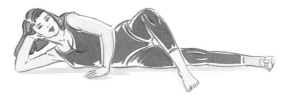

2 Bend your left knee, placing your foot flat on the floor in front of the right leg. Flex your right foot and extend the leg so the inner thigh faces the ceiling.

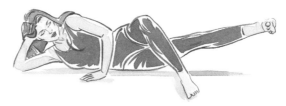

3 Pull in your stomach, contract your inner thigh, and lift the right leg up about 10cm (4in). Hold for 5 seconds and lower. Repeat 10 times. Change legs and repeat.

TOP TIPS

■ Cellulite particularly affects the inner thigh area. To combat it, check out the information in Beating Cellulite on pages 116–17.

■ Pliés are excellent leg and buttock toners. To make them even more effective, squeeze your inner thighs and buttock muscles as you raise yourself up. There are more ballet-style exercises on page 102.

■ You can work your inner thighs while sitting in front of the television or at a computer. Put a pillow between your knees, squeeze hard, and release. Repeat as many times as you can, as often as you can.

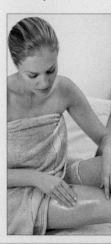

OUTER THIGH TONE

The outer thighs are a major problem area for many women. Make yours look leaner and more shapely by doing the Total-body Warm-up (p88), then tackling these three simple exercises. Stand on a non-slip surface for the outer thigh lift. Use a mat or towel to lie on for the other exercises. Even if the size of your thighs doesn't reduce, they will soon look much more toned.

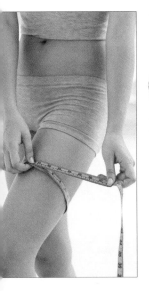

OUTER THIGH LIFT

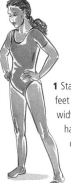

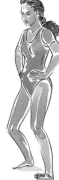

1 Stand with your feet shoulder-width apart and hands on a chair or your hip bones. Lift your left leg out to the side keeping your foot flexed. Hold for a count of five. Return to starting position.

2 Slowly bend your knees, as though you are going to sit down on a low stool. Raise your left leg forwards a little off the ground and hold the stretch for a count of five. Repeat the exercise 10 times on each leg.

OUTER THIGH RAISE

1 Lie on your right side, propped up on your right forearm, leaning slightly forwards and with your legs bent at a 45-degree angle.

2 Raise your left leg, keeping it parallel to the ceiling, using the outer thigh muscle to do the work. Return to starting position. Repeat 10 times on each leg.

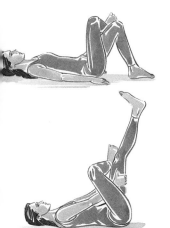

OUTER THIGH STRETCH

1 Lie flat on your back with your knees bent, feet flat on the floor, and your hands palms-down by your sides. Lift your left leg and rest your ankle on your right thigh, just above the knee. You should feel the stretch along the outer edge of your left thigh.

2 For a bigger stretch, lift your right leg as high as you can, supporting your right thigh with both hands. Keep your head as close to the floor as possible and keep your back flat on the floor. Pull your right leg in gently until you feel the stretch in your left thigh. Use your right leg to push the left leg forwards to stretch the outer thigh and gluteal (buttock) muscles. Hold for a count of five. Repeat 10 times on both legs.

TOP TIPS

■ To see quick results, do these exercises once or twice daily.

■ Do toning exercises at a variety of tempos – ultraslow and then pulsing more quickly – to get the maximum benefit from the movements.

■ Build up the number of repetitions slowly. You might not be able to do the whole routine at the first attempt. After doing the routine regularly for a few weeks, however, you'll find that you are up to the suggested number of repetitions. Then you can add more, making sure you are listening to your body all the time to be certain you aren't putting it under any strain.

■ Firm up your whole lower body by following up these exercises with those outlined in Inner Thigh Tone on page 96 and Better Buttocks on page 95.

■ Aerobic exercise, such as dancing, running, power-walking, rowing, swimming or cycling, will help keep your lower body in trim, too.

LEANER LEGS

Legs get a workout whenever you walk or use the stairs instead of an elevator. There are, however, useful targeted exercises you can do to make your legs shapelier. March in place for a few minutes to warm up before starting. You will need a wall for support, a mat or towel to lie on, and, if you want to add to the effectiveness of the moves, tin cans or bottles of water to use as weights.

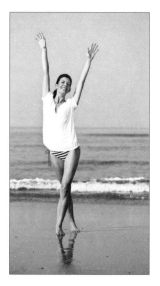

BEND AND STRAIGHTEN

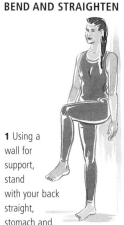

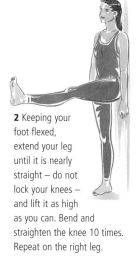

1 Using a wall for support, stand with your back straight, stomach and buttocks pulled in. Lift your left knee until your thigh forms a right angle with your calf.

2 Keeping your foot flexed, extend your leg until it is nearly straight – do not lock your knees – and lift it as high as you can. Bend and straighten the knee 10 times. Repeat on the right leg.

THIGH PRESS AND LIFT

Lie on your side with your head supported on your hand, elbow on the floor. Pull your abdominals in. Bend your lower leg slightly and keep the top leg straight and in line with your hip and shoulder. Flex your foot and point your toes down. Use your outer thigh muscle to lift your top leg about 2.5cm (1in) above the line of your hip. Lower to the floor. Repeat 10 times, then change sides.

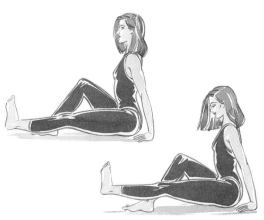

FRONT OF LEG SHAPE

1 Sit on the floor with your left leg bent, the right leg flat on the floor. Place your hands behind your buttocks with palms flat on the floor. Lean against a wall if you need extra support for your back.

2 Hold in your abdominal muscles and extend the right leg, with foot flexed and toes pointing towards the ceiling. Then slowly raise it about 5–7cm (2–3cm) off the floor and lower it. Repeat 10 times and change legs.

TOP TIPS

■ To give calves and ankles a workout, try to walk around barefoot as much as you can. Walking barefoot on sand is especially beneficial for shaping your leg muscles.

■ If you suffer from puffy ankles in the heat or because you have to stand a lot, rotate your ankles several times in both directions to reduce the swelling. This also helps to reduce puffiness when you're travelling by air, too.

■ Walking is great exercise for the legs and puts less strain on the body than jogging, making it more accessible if you are very unfit or have problems with your joints. Check out the information on Power-walking on page 80.

■ The shins of the legs contain no sebaceous (oil-producing) glands, which is why you tend to have dry skin around this area. To help improve the look and feel of your legs, see the exfoliating techniques on page 114 and the moisturizing tips on page 119.

CHEST EXERCISES

The majority of women want a firm, toned bust. Exercise cannot make the bust bigger because there is no muscle in the breasts, but you can firm up the surrounding area and give your breasts extra support and lift. Warm up by marching in place for a couple of minutes. You will need a mat or towel to lie on, and light weights or cans of food.

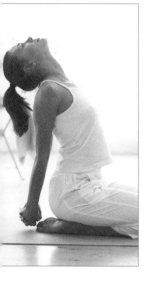

ELBOW PRESS

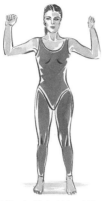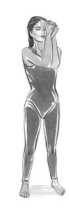

1 Stand with feet hip-width apart, knees slightly bent, arms raised out to the sides. Keep your elbows bent and your hands in soft 'fists.'

2 Bring elbows and forearms in so they are pressing together in front of your chest. Hold for 5 seconds. Repeat up to 10 times.

PALM CLASPS

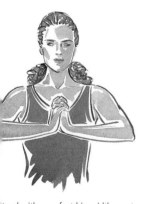

Stand with your feet hip-width apart or sit up straight in your chair if you want to do it at your desk. Place the palms of your hands together in front of your chest with your fingers interlinked. Pull in and tighten your abdominal muscles. Press your palms together hard and hold for 5 seconds. Repeat the exercise up to 10 times in each session.

ELBOW CROSSES

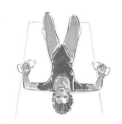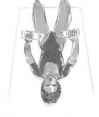

1 Lie on your back, knees bent, feet flat on the floor, holding the weights with your elbows bent.

2 Push your hands up towards the ceiling, palms facing forwards towards your thighs.

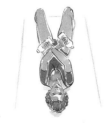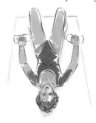

3 Slowly move your arms towards each other, so that your elbows cross above your chest.

4 Slowly lower your arms. Repeat up to 10 times, alternating the arm crossing over at the top.

WAIST WORKSHOP

Weight and extra inches go on to the waist all too easily as we get older if we lead a sedentary lifestyle that doesn't burn off the calories we consume. Fortunately, it's also easy to trim your waist with a combination of a low-fat diet and a simple sequence of exercises. You will need a mat or towel to lie on and tin cans or bottles of water to use as weights.

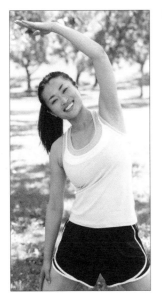

SIDE STRETCHES

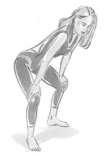

1 First warm up the lower back (see Spine Thrillers p107). Bend forwards 30 degrees, placing your hands above your kneecaps to support your back. Round out gently, then straighten your spine eight times.

2 Stand with feet hip-width apart, arms by your sides. Stretch your right arm slowly down your side towards your right ankle. Return to the starting position. Stretch your left arm towards your left ankle. Do 10 stretches on each side. Lift the other arm above your head for a deeper stretch. Build up to more reps and using weights.

SIDE TWIST

1 Lie on your back, pressing your lower back firmly into the floor and tightening your stomach muscles. Raise your legs straight up in front of you, keeping the knees slightly bent. Stretch towards your left foot with your right hand, then towards your right foot with your left hand. Use your abdominals, not your neck or back, to do the work. Reach up to alternate sides 20 times (10 on each side). Rest for 5 seconds and try another set of 20 'reaches'.

2 Lie on your back with your knees bent. Put your right foot on your left knee. Place your left hand under your head at the nape of your neck. Hold in your abdominals, lift up and twist to the right, leading with your shoulder not your elbow. Return to the starting position. Repeat on the other side. Do 10 repetitions on each side.

3 Lie on your back with your knees bent, feet on the floor, your arms down by your sides and your fingertips pointing towards your toes. Contract your abdominals and raise your head and shoulders slightly off the floor. Continue to contract your stomach muscles and push your right hand towards your right foot. Repeat on the other side. Alternate up to 10 times.

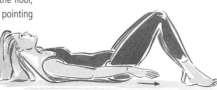

TOP TIPS

■ Choose clothes carefully to highlight your good physical features and disguise problem areas. If you don't have a well-defined waist, for example, looser, low-slung trousers are more flattering. Avoid pleated trousers as these emphasize the waist area; instead go for flat-fronted styles with a chunky belt. Fitted shirts and jackets that are nipped in at the waist help give the illusion of a slim waist, but don't try pulling yourself in with wide belts – they usually emphasize a lack of waist.

■ Improving the muscle tone of your shoulders and upper body will help define your waist. Try doing the Super Shoulders routine on page 93. Add a weekly swim to your fitness and exercise routine to supplement this upper body workout.

■ Once you are used to doing Side Stretches, start to hold light weights in both hands while you do the stretches and up the number of repetitions you do at every session.

TONED STOMACH

Unlike leg and arm muscles, the abdominal muscles get little exercise in the course of a normal day. For this reason the stomach can quickly become slack and untoned. Women tend to store weight around the stomach, making the problem worse. The good news is that abdominal muscles respond well to exercise. With just a few targeted routines, you can quickly tone up your tummy.

STOMACH CURL

1 Lie on the floor with feet hip-width apart and your knees bent. Keep your back flat against the floor, tighten your stomach muscles and gently raise your head and shoulders a few inches. Keep your chin off your chest throughout the exercise.

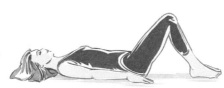

2 Slide your hands as far up towards your knees as you can, hold for a few seconds, then slowly return to the starting position. Repeat 10 times, keeping the movement smooth, not jerky. As this exercise becomes easier, work up to 40 repetitions.

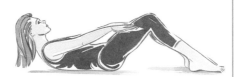

LOWER ABDOMEN CURL

1 Lie on the floor with your knees bent, feet hip-width apart and your lower back pressed into the ground. Put your arms, palms down, by your sides.

2 Raise your legs off the floor up into the air and contract your stomach to lift your buttocks towards the ceiling, then lower them. Repeat 10 times and work up to 40 repetitions. Keep your legs bent to make the exercise easier.

CRUNCH TIME

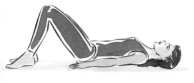

1 Lie on your back, knees bent and hip-width apart, feet on the floor. Tighten your stomach muscles and press your back firmly into the floor.

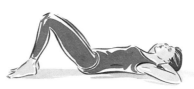

2 Place your hands loosely by the sides of your temples, with your elbows out to the sides. Keep your chin up – as if you have a small ball under it.

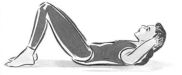

3 Keeping your neck straight and your chin lifted, exhale and use your tightened stomach muscles to curl up towards your knees, until your shoulder blades are off the floor.

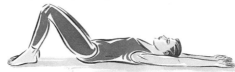

4 Inhale and lower yourself gently, keeping your back pressed firmly into the floor. Repeat 10 times and work up to 40 repetitions as this exercise becomes easier. Then stretch out your arms.

TOP TIPS

■ If you suffer from minor back aches and pains, weak abdominal muscles may be the cause. Do these stomach toning exercises at least three times a week to strengthen your stomach muscles. They will help improve poor posture, too. If you have back problems, always get professional medical advice before starting a new exercise programme.

■ As you become more familiar with the exercises you will be able to start controlling your breathing to make them more effective. For all these stomach exercises, breathe out as you lift your body and breathe in as you lower it.

■ It is important to hold your stomach muscles in as you do crunches – imagine your belly button is pressing down into your spine.

■ If your back does feel uncomfortable after exercise – or after carrying shopping or just sitting at a desk all day – try the Spine Thrillers on page 107 or Essential Relaxation on p108.

BALLET STYLE

Dancers' bodies always look lean, strong and incredibly graceful. Dancers also move with great poise and have excellent posture. Try these simple movements based on ballet exercises to make your body stronger and more flexible and help improve your posture. If you enjoy them, why not see if there are any ballet classes in your local area – it's a great way to tone up and get fit.

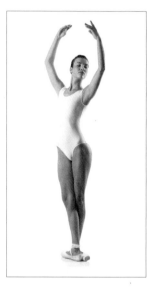

EXTENDED PLIÉ

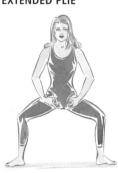 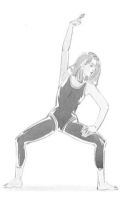

1 Stand with your feet apart, toes pointing out and arms in front of your body. Contract your stomach and buttocks. Bend your knees and lower your body, keeping your knees above your heels.

2 Place your left hand on your left thigh and lean to the left. Extend your right arm over your head. Hold in place for 20 seconds. Repeat five times on each side.

BALLETIC STRETCH

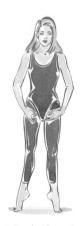

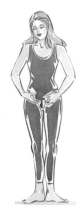

DEMI-PLIÉ

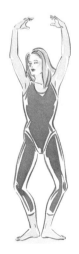

1 Stand with your heels together, toes pointing out, arms in front of you held at hip level. Breathe in, then breathe out as you tighten your abdominals and buttocks, and rise on to the balls of your feet.

2 Extend your arms overhead, keeping your shoulders down and relaxed. Breathe in as you slowly release your feet back down to the floor. Repeat the exercise up to 10 times.

1 Stand with your heels together, toes pointing out, arms held loosely in front of you at hip level. Breathe in and bend your knees, keeping your feet flat on the floor.

2 Extend your arms gracefully overhead. Breathe out and squeeze your buttocks and thighs as you slowly return to standing. Repeat this exercise 10 times.

TOP TIPS

■ In all these ballet-style exercises, make sure that your weight is evenly distributed through your feet and that you are able to wiggle your toes, indicating that your feet are relaxed.

■ Do these exercises in front of a mirror from time to time so that you can check your posture and the alignment of your body.

■ If you find it hard to balance on tiptoe, concentrate on looking at a fixed, still point in front of you.

■ T'ai Chi is an exercise programme that employs a similar graceful and tranquil style. If you enjoy ballet-style exercises, you might also enjoy this eastern form of exercise. Check out what classes are available in your area.

■ Stretching exercises, such as Stretch Slimmer opposite and Stretch It Out on page 105 combine well with these ballet exercises if you want to extend the routine. You could finish with Essential Relaxaton on page 108.

STRETCH SLIMMER

To help you lengthen shortened muscles and loosen tight ones, try these simple stretches. They are ideal if your body has become rather inflexible through lack of exercise. So if touching your toes has become a distant memory, get stretching! You will notice an improvement surprisingly quickly. The other good news is that you will develop a longer, leaner, trimmer body.

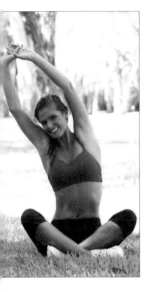

SHOULDER STRETCH

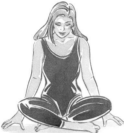

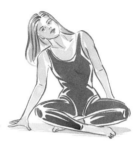

1 Sit on the floor with your legs crossed comfortably in front of you. Tilt your head forwards slightly. Spread out your fingers on the floor by your sides for support. Breathe regularly and evenly.

2 Look straight ahead and tilt your head gently to the right. Feel the stretch in your neck. Rotate your left shoulder clockwise and then counter-clockwise. Repeat the action on the other side.

SIDE STRETCHES

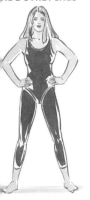

LOWER BODY STRETCH

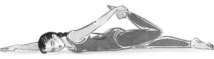

1 Lie on your front and turn your head sideways, relax your shoulders and point your right arm forwards. Bend your left knee and hold at the ankle with your left hand. Ease your leg into the buttock. Feel the stretch in the hip and thigh. Hold the pose for 20 seconds and then change legs.

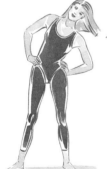

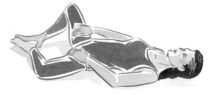

1 Stand with your feet shoulder-width apart, your knees soft and slightly bent. Keep your hands on your waist and your hips and legs still throughout the exercise for maximum effect. Breathe steadily and fairly deeply.

2 Bend your upper body to the left slowly and gently. Keep the movement controlled. Return to upright, then bend to the right, feeling the stretch in your waist. Return to upright. Repeat the stretch up to 10 times.

2 Lie on your back and make a diamond shape with your legs – soles of feet together and knees dropping out to your sides as shown above. Hold the pose for 20 seconds. Apply a little pressure with your hands to your inner thighs to increase the stretch. Relax and repeat up to 10 times.

TOP TIPS

■ Combining a stretching routine with aerobic activity will increase the effectiveness of both activities. You will find you can stretch much further after you have exercised and your muscles are warm. Stretching also prevents muscular aches and pains after you've worked your muscles hard aerobically.

■ Aches and pains when you wake up are not simply a natural sign of aging. They are also due to tension collecting in the muscles. Mental stress, as well as unusual physical exertion, is usually the cause of tension. You may not notice it during the day while you are moving around, but it can accumulate during sleep. The key to avoiding morning aches is to stretch out before you go to bed. This relaxes your mind and your body. Check out the Stretch It Out exercises on page 105 and the Essential Relaxation routine on page 108. You can also stretch out very gently in bed before you get up, but be aware that your muscles will be cold.

MINIMAL MOVES

Some fitness experts believe that the best, and most effective, type of exercise is small, controlled movements that tone the muscles deep down. Bear in mind that you need to make a lot of tiny controlled movements for maximum results. You will need a mat or towel to lie on and a firm chair for support during this routine.

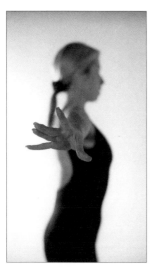

HIPS, BUTTOCKS AND THIGHS TIGHTENER

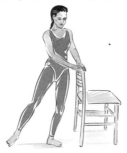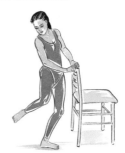

1 Stand with feet together, hands resting on the back of a chair. Take your right leg out to the side, flexing your foot and pointing your toes towards the floor. Bend your left knee.

2 Move your hips to the left slightly, bring your right leg in and tighten your buttocks. Move your right leg up and down just 5mm (¼in). Repeat 25 times, then do the other side.

SHOULDER PRESSES

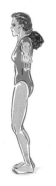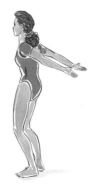

1 Stand erect, feet hip-width apart. Bend your knees slightly. Take your arms up and out to the side, keeping them straight and in line with your shoulders. Slowly rotate your hands backwards so your palms and thumbs face the ceiling. Tighten your buttocks and abdomen.

2 Curl your pelvis up. Move your arms behind your back, keeping your hands roughly level with your shoulders and arms straight. With tiny movements move your arms 5mm (¼in) upwards. Repeat at least 25 times, and build up to 50.

STOMACH TIGHTENER

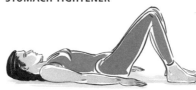

1 Lie on the floor with your knees bent, feet hip-width apart, arms by your sides. Breathe out and gradually curl up, using your stomach muscles to lift you and raise your head and shoulders off the floor. Do not arch your back.

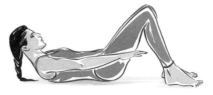

2 Keeping your stomach tight and head raised, lift your arms 15cm (6in) off the floor. In slow motion move your hands 5mm (¼in) towards your feet and then back again. Repeat this tiny movement 25 times and aim for 50 repetitions.

TOP TIPS

■ The slow, controlled movements described here require a great deal of concentration. Think very carefully about the muscle you are working as you do each exercise to help make the movements as effective as possible, and imagine you are pushing your limbs through a thick, viscous liquid. Try to keep your breathing smooth and even and your movements slow, controlled and fluid.

■ Make the shoulder presses harder by holding light weights.

■ Slow exercises that isolate particular muscle groups, also called isometric exercises, can help you to build lean muscle strength relatively quickly if you practice the movements at least three times a week.

■ Having good posture – head held high, body erect, yet relaxed – can help you to look stronger, leaner, and firmer. The exercises on this page will help you become more conscious of your muscle strength and to improve your posture.

STRETCH IT OUT

Muscular tension is the body's natural response to stress. The shoulders, neck and lower back tend to be the most stress-prone sites. This simple series of stretches targets the tension hotspots in your body and are a good cool-down after aerobic exercise or stretching and toning. Use a mat or towel to lie on to provide a soft surface beneath your spine.

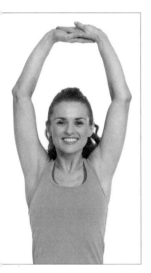

LEG LIGHTENER

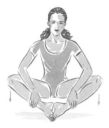

1 Sit cross-legged with your back straight. Bend your legs in front of you and press the soles of your feet together. Hold on to your ankles and use your elbows to press your thighs and knees down towards the floor. Hold for 20 seconds. Repeat.

2 Lie on your back. Bend your knees so your feet are flat on the floor. Raise your left leg to your chest, holding it behind the calf. Stretch (make sure you do not straighten) the raised leg and pull it towards you. Hold for 10–20 seconds. Relax. Change legs.

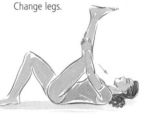

FULL BODY STRETCH

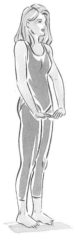
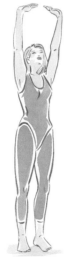
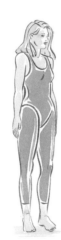

1 Stand with your feet slightly apart, legs straight but not locked, hands in front of you at the tops of your thighs, with fingers pointing towards each other and palms down.

2 Move your arms forwards and upwards, inhaling through your nose. Hold your arms above your head, pushing palms upwards, pulling your elbows close to your ears.

3 Hold the stretch and breathe out through your mouth. Slowly lower your arms to your sides. Repeat the steps 10 times and build up to more repetitions as you get more practised.

STRETCH THEN RELAX

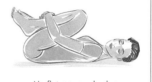

Lie flat on your back on the floor, looking at the ceiling, and bring your knees into your chest. Wrap your arms around your legs for support. Gently roll your head to the right, then bring it very slowly back to the starting position. Let your head roll to the left. Bring it slowly back to centre. Put your feet on the floor and slowly slide your legs out straight. Put your arms at your side, palms up. Relax fully for 5 minutes, breathing slowly, evenly and deeply.

TOP TIPS

■ If you have time, warm up before you start the stress-relieving stretches on this page. March in place, run up and down the stairs or dance for a few minutes. This will raise your body temperature and help release any pent-up stress or anger.

■ Breathe slowly as you perform each stretch, breathing in through your nostrils, pausing before you breathe out, then slowly releasing all the air in your lungs and pausing before filling your lungs with air again. As you do each stretch, keep telling yourself you are relaxing and slowing down.

■ Firm feet will allow the rest of your body to relax and move more freely. When standing, keep your weight on your heels so you can spread your toes out wide and the arches of your feet feel strong and springy. This allows your spine to straighten and lengthen. Relax your shoulders and arms and imagine a strong thread pulling up through your spine and the top of your head.

BACK BASICS

Joints rely on movement for lubrication, and ligaments and muscles tighten and tense if they are not stretched regularly. Exercising and stretching your back frequently will help prevent everyday aches and pains as well as making you more supple. You will need a mat or towel to lie on, and tin cans or bottles of water to use as weights.

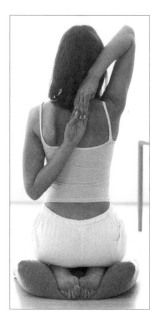

SHOULDERS AND UPPER BACK

1 Stand with knees relaxed, palms facing your thighs. Bring your shoulders back and squeeze the shoulder blades and upper back muscles together as you move your hands around and up from your thighs to the sides of your hips.

2 With your shoulders still back, shrug them as close to your ears as you can. Release and bring your hands back to your thighs. Repeat this movement at least 10 times. Use light weights to increase the exercise's effectiveness.

TOP TIPS

■ For a simple back and shoulder stretch that can be done anywhere, reach one arm down your back, towards the middle and clasp the fingers of that hand, by bending up your other arm from the bottom, as shown in the photograph. Hold the position for a slow count of 10, then repeat using opposite arms.

■ Do not bounce or force stretches. If a limb starts to shake as you stretch it, you have pushed it too far. You should feel the tension, but there shouldn't be any pain.

■ If you work at a computer, position it directly in front of you and have your chair adjusted to the correct height for the desk so that your legs bend at right angles at the knee.

STRETCH OUT

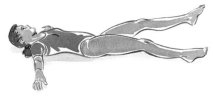

1 Lie on your back with your arms outstretched at shoulder level. Tighten your abdominal muscles. Raise your left leg slowly.

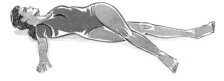

2 Move your left leg across the right leg. Keep your shoulders and back pressed into the floor. Hold the pose for 5 seconds. Repeat with other leg. Do the sequence five times on each side.

A STRONGER SPINE

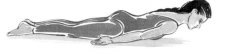

1 Lie face down, arms by your sides and close to body, forehead touching the floor. Raise your head and shoulders. Hold for 5 seconds. Repeat, with your hands behind your head. Hold for 5 seconds and relax. Do not raise your head and shoulders any higher than is comfortable.

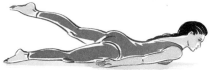

2 Raise your head and shoulders and each leg in turn, hold for 5 seconds, and then relax. Repeat the sequence five times.

TAKE CARE

These exercises are not intended for those suffering from chronic back pain. Prior to starting them, see your doctor or a back specialist for advice. If any of these exercises cause any pain, stop doing them immediately.

SPINE THRILLERS

These stretches may be familiar to you if you have ever been to a yoga class. Yoga is the perfect antidote to stress, combining as it does mental tranquility with physical fitness and spiritual awareness. Try these gentle poses, which have been specially selected to ease and strengthen your back and are ideal for doing after swimming, which uses many of the muscles in your back.

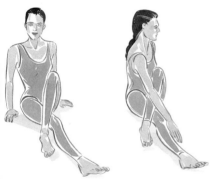

CAT STRETCH

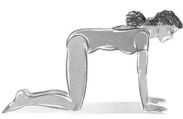

1 Get down on all fours, hands positioned directly underneath your shoulders, hips over your knees. Breathe slowly and evenly, trying to make your back as level as possible. Let your head and neck relax down.

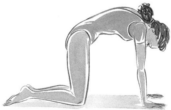

2 Slowly push your spine up towards the ceiling, tucking your chin into your chest. Feel a stretch along your spine and shoulders. Do not push the stretch if you feel any discomfort. Hold for 10 seconds.

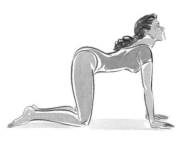

3 Slowly bring your head up and push your spine down so your back is as concave as possible. Hold for about 10 seconds, then make your back level and relax your head and neck. Repeat the sequence several times.

THE SPINE TWIST

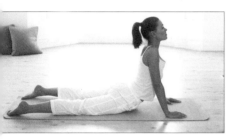

Sit with your legs stretched out in front of you, palms on the floor. Lift your left leg and place the foot on the far side of your right knee. Slowly turn your body to the left and reach towards your right ankle with your right hand.

2 Place your left hand behind you, palm down, trying to keep your back straight. Each time you breathe out, twist further to the left. Stop when you feel stretched and hold for 10 seconds. Relax then repeat on the other side.

COBRA

Lie on your stomach with your forehead on the floor. Put your hands palms down under your shoulders. Push your arms up and stretch your head up. Hold the pose for 10 seconds, then relax down. Repeat the movement several times.

TOP TIPS

■ If you enjoy stretching and calming exercises, look for a local yoga class to attend. It is an ideal form of exercise for all ages and fitness levels.

■ Stretch out and move around as much as possible during the day. This will stop tension from accumulating in your spine. Slumping at your desk, long periods of sitting down, poor posture and feeling stressed can all take their toll on your back, so get stretching!

■ In yoga, breathing is considered the life-force of an individual's being, affecting emotional and spiritual harmony. Breathe evenly and deeply throughout the stretches. Concentrate on breathing out for longer than you breathe in since this will help you to relax and focus more.

TAKE CARE

Do not push yourself into any position that feels uncomfortable or where you might lose your balance. If at any point you feel dizzy or faint, stop and relax.

ESSENTIAL RELAXATION

Relaxation is a skill. You have to learn how to do it and you need to practise regularly. The only equipment you need for this routine are comfortable clothes and a towel or mat to lie on. Aim to do the relaxer several times a week – when you get home from work, after a journey or before bed. It is also beneficial to do this sequence after stretching or working out.

REST AND RESTORE ROUTINE

1 Lie on your back in a quiet, dimly lit room. Close your eyes. Let your feet flop outwards and your arms fall away from the body, palms facing the ceiling.

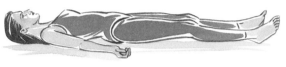

Breathe deeply and gently. Concentrate on your chest rising and falling as you breathe in and out. Make an effort to slow your breathing down. Screw up your face muscles, then relax them. Imagine that your skin is so relaxed that all the lines on your face are ironed out and your skin is slipping down towards the floor.

2 Press your shoulders into the floor. Hold for 10 seconds, relax and repeat. Lift your head off the floor without straining your neck, lengthen the back of the neck and gently put your head down. Check your jaw and neck muscles are relaxed.

3 Stretch your arms and fingers out above you. Hold the stretch for about 10 seconds. Relax and let your arms and hands fall gently back to the floor.

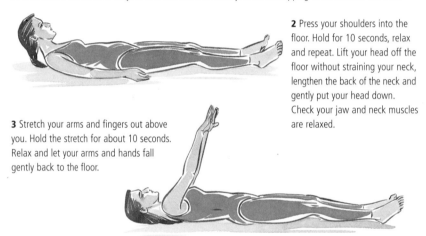

4 Hold in your stomach and lift your buttocks off the floor, without straining your lower back, then let them back down. Feel your spine stretch gently and relax. Keeping your legs together, stretch your legs and toes. Hold for 10 seconds, then relax, letting your feet fall open. If any part of your body still feels tense, repeat the sequence.

5 Stay in this relaxed pose for up to 10 minutes. Concentrate on your breathing whenever day-to-day worries enter your mind. Before you get up, roll on to your side and stay there for a minute. Get up slowly as your blood pressure may be low.

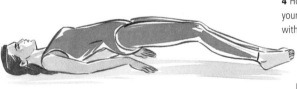

TOP TIPS

■ A traditional relaxation pose is shown here, but some people find it uncomfortable to lie flat on the floor. You could try the sequence lying on your bed or put down a thick blanket.

■ You may find you get cold quickly when you are fully relaxed. Have a throw or blanket handy to pull over you. You need to be warm to relax fully.

■ To help combat tension even more, burn a relaxing aromatherapy oil such as lavender or chamomile while you do relaxation routines.

■ A daily form of complete physical and mental relaxation will clear your mind and help to relieve recurrent backaches and headaches. It can also lower blood pressure and keep a number of physical complaints at bay.

■ Doing these exercises after vigorous activity in the evening can counteract the adrenalin from aerobic exercise and help you to sleep.

FACIAL WORKOUT

Your face can benefit from exercise too. Toning your facial muscles can help prevent sagging, improve circulation and skin tone, and reduce double chins and puffy, baggy eyes. Do these simple exercises for a few minutes twice a day as part of your beauty and exercise regime and you will see positive results in just a few weeks.

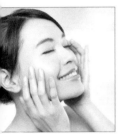

SCULPTURED CHEEKS

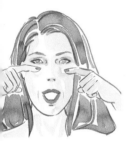

Position your index fingers on top of each cheekbone. Open your mouth, pushing the top and bottom lips apart to form a long 'O' shape.

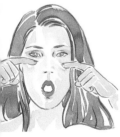

Hold the 'O' shape, keeping your upper lip pressed against the top teeth. Smile with the corners of your mouth and release. Repeat slowly five times, feeling the cheek muscles move and work.

EYE OPENERS

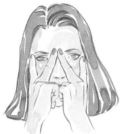

1 Place your middle fingers gently between your eyebrows, just above the bridge of the nose. Position your index fingers lightly at the outer corners of your eyes.

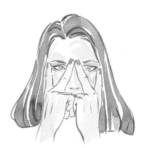

2 Roll your eyes up and look at an imaginary line down the centre of your forehead. Repeat and release 10 times. Keep looking up and in and squeeze your eyelids shut for a count of 40.

A DEFINED CHIN

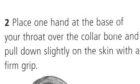

1 Sit up straight with your chin held high. Close your lips tightly together and try to smile using only your upper lip.

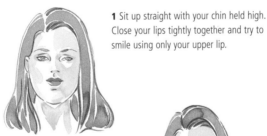

2 Place one hand at the base of your throat over the collar bone and pull down slightly on the skin with a firm grip.

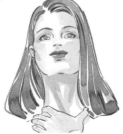

3 Tilt your head back gently and you will feel a strong pull on the chin and neck muscles. Return your head to the starting position and repeat steps 2 and 3 around 30 times.

TOP TIPS

■ Make these exercises part of your daily skin-cleansing routine – you'll be able to see what you're doing in the mirror. Alternatively, when you have mastered the techniques and can do the exercises without a mirror, you can do the routine while relaxing in the bath or even at your desk when everyone is out at lunch!

■ Another quick exercise to work your face is to raise your eyebrows as high as they will go, keeping the rest of your face still. Hold for a count of five lower, and repeat for about 1 minute.

■ Feeding your skin with the right nutrients will improve its condition, so a healthy diet will soon improve the look of your skin. 'Water' your skin by drinking six to eight glasses of water a day, too.

■ Too-rapid weight loss can make your face look older, as there is less fat to plump out the wrinkles. Try to stay at a healthy weight and don't go below the ideal BMI. Being too thin for your natural frame is neither healthy nor especially attractive.

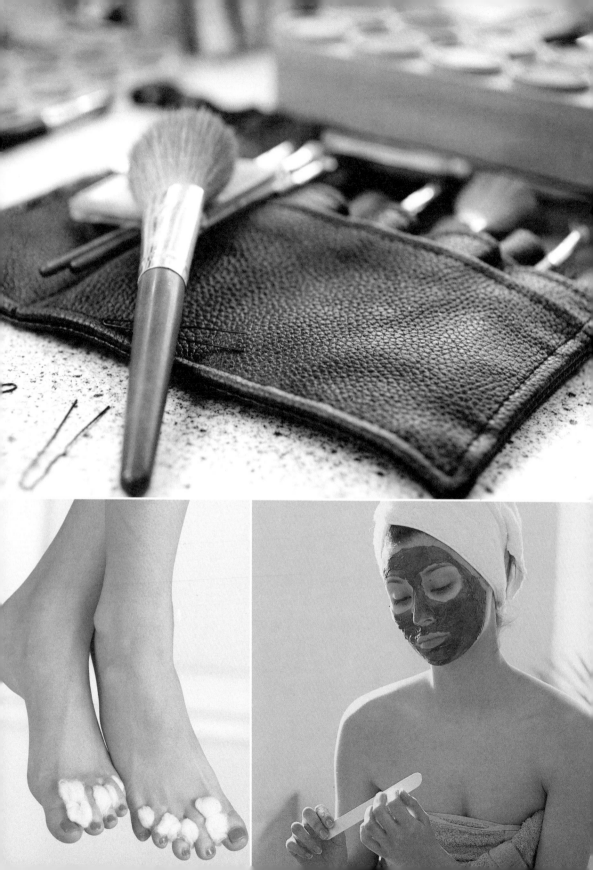

COMPLETE BODYCARE

The secret to a beautiful-looking body is
to lavish the same care on it as you do
on your complexion and make-up. You
need to take into account general
maintenance and any requirements it
may have. Whatever beauty boosts
your body needs, you'll find the help you
need in this section of the book.

BATHROOM ESSENTIALS

A pleasing, well-stocked bathroom can make all the difference at the start of a busy day and can be transformed into a sensual haven to help you unwind at the end of it. There is a huge range of products available, but actually you only really need a few simple items.

The skin is the body's largest organ and forms a protective barrier against bacteria and other invaders. Although it continually sheds and renews itself, the skin has a lot to cope with and it deserves special attention. Scrubbing our skin removes dead skin cells and stimulates the blood supply, leaving skin tingling and toned. So keeping clean is vital for the overall health of the skin and body.

SPONGES AND FACECLOTHS
These are useful for lathering soaps and gels on your skin, and dislodging dirt and grime from your body. Wash your facecloth regularly and allow it to dry between uses. Natural sponges are a more expensive but long-lasting alternative. Squeeze out afterwards in warm water and allow to dry naturally.

PUMICE STONE
These are made from very porous volcanic rock and work best if you lather up with soap before rubbing at

Right Bathing can be one of life's most pleasurable necessities.

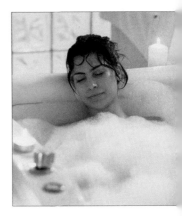

hardened areas of skin in a circular motion. Don't rub too fiercely or you'll make the skin sore. A 'little and often' approach is best.

LOOFAH OR BACK BRUSH
Try using a loofah as an exfoliator as its length makes it useful for scrubbing difficult-to-reach areas such as the back. Loofahs are actually the pod of an Egyptian plant and need a bit of care if they're going to last. Rinse and drain them thoroughly after use to prevent them going black and mouldy. Avoid rinsing them in vinegar and lemon juice as this can be too harsh for these once-living things.

Back brushes are also useful for areas of skin that are hard to reach, and are easier to care for: you simply rinse them in cool water after use and leave them to dry.

SOAPS AND CLEANSING BARS
These are a cheap and effective way of cleansing your body. If you find them too drying, choose ones that contain moisturizing ingredients to minimize these effects. Most people can use ordinary soaps and cleansers without any problem. However, if you have very dry or sensitive skin, it is advisable to opt for the pH-balanced variety.

BATHROOM BASICS
From cleaning your teeth to preventing underarm odour, there are a few basics that are essential for any bathroom:
• **Toothbrush:** It is vital to choose the right toothbrush. A nylon brush is best, as bristle ones split and lose their shape quickly. Choose one with a small head so you can easily clean your back teeth. A soft or medium brush is best as harder brushes may damage the tooth enamel and gums. Change your toothbrush about every month.
• **Dental floss:** Use floss at least once a day to clean between the teeth where the toothbrush can't reach. Waxed floss is best as it's less likely to catch on fillings or uneven edges. To floss, wind a

short length around the second finger of each hand. Slide it gently down between two of the teeth, taking care to press it against the side of the tooth. Then gently slide it upwards out of the teeth, removing any food particles with it. Repeat between all of the teeth.
• **Antiperspirant deodorant:** Deodorants do not prevent perspiration – they only stop the bacteria from decomposing the sweat. If you perspire heavily, it is advisable to use an antiperspirant or, even better, an antiperspirant deodorant, since the antiperspirant element prevents the production of sweat. However, remember not to use it on inflamed or broken skin or immediately after shaving.

• **Talcum powder:** This white powder is made from finely ground magnesium silicate and is usually perfumed. It is considered to be rather old-fashioned, which is a shame because a good talcum powder makes you smell fresh and helps you slide into your clothes. However, there is no substitute for drying with a towel, especially between the toes, for keeping your skin healthy.

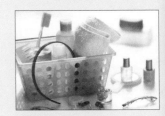

CARING FOR YOUR BODY

egular pampering may seem like an indulgence but in fact taking care of your whole body is vital keeping it healthy. The power of touch to identify problem areas and notice changes, as you noisturize, scrub and massage, should not be underestimated.

ne of the most effective ways to care for ur body is to build bodycare treatments to your everyday bathroom routine. ands and feet, elbows and necks can be rgotten and neglected because we are t in the habit of focusing our attention h them. The next time you are in the bath shower, make a quick assessment and sk yourself the following questions:

HROAT
Does skincare stop at your neck?
Is the skin rough and grey?
Do you regularly indulge yourself
with special treats to keep your skin
in tip-top condition?

HEST
Do you give your breasts the care
they need?
Is your chest prone to break-outs?
Do you protect this area of your skin
from the harmful rays of the sun?

RMS
Are your elbows grey and dull in tone?
Is the skin soft and supple, or rough
and dry?

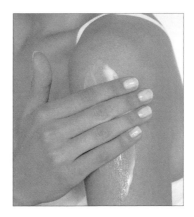

Above The tops and the backs of arms need care too, so that they stay soft, smooth and firm.

- Do darker hairs on your lower arms
  need bleaching?
- If you remove hair from your
  underarms, have you found the best
  method, the one that suits you for
  convenience and results?
- Have you found the solution to
  underarm freshness?
- Do you exfoliate the back of your arms?

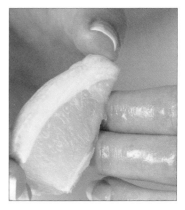

Above The juice of a lemon is a good natural bleach for nails that have been stained by dark nail polish.

HANDS
- Do your hands suffer from doing too
  much housework?
- Do they need some moisturizing care?
- Are your nails neatly filed and shaped?
- Would a lick of polish or a French
  manicure give them a helping hand?

LEGS
- Are they free from stubbly hairs?
- Is the skin as smooth as it could be?
- Would they benefit from fake tan?
- Are they prone to cellulite?
- Would bathtime treats improve the
  look of your skin?

BIKINI LINE
- If you remove hair from this area, have
  you found the best method for you?

FEET
- Are they free from hard skin, corns
  and calluses?
- Are your nails neatly trimmed?
- Do you smooth a foot cream on them
  regularly to ensure that the skin
  stays soft?

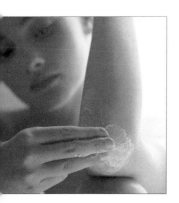

bove Remember to exfoliate the skin on ur elbows, as this is often overlooked and n become dry.

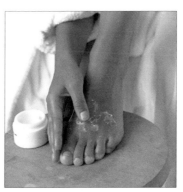

Above As you massage your feet, apply cream to the soles of your feet, as the skin on the heels can become dry and cracked.

BE A SMOOTHIE

Most women aspire to smooth, healthy skin free of dry patches, superfluous hair and blemishes. And the chances are, even if your skin isn't prone to spottiness or flaky patches, it will suffer from dullness and poor condition from time to time.

Body scrubs and exfoliators are the answer to rough skin. They work by shifting dead cells from the skin surface, revealing the younger, fresher ones underneath. This process also stimulates the circulation of blood in the skin tissues, giving it a glow.

Hair on a woman's body is completely natural, but fashion and cultural practices mean that it is usually removed. There are a number of ways of removing hair for smooth, soft skin and it is simply a matter of finding the method that suits you best.

EXFOLIATION METHODS

There are lots of different ways you can exfoliate your body – so there's one to suit every budget and preference.
• Your first option is to buy an exfoliating scrub, which is a cream- or gel-based product containing tiny abrasive particles. Look for the type with rounded particles that won't irritate delicate skin. Simply massage the scrub into damp skin, then rinse away with lots of warm water.

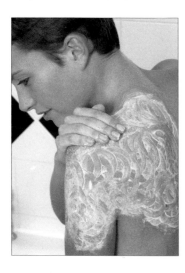

Above A body scrub is a quick and easy way to keep your skin sleek and smooth.

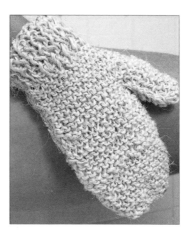

Above Keep a sisal mitt to hand for really super-soft skin.

• Bath mitts, loofahs and sisal mitts are a cinch to use, and cost-effective too. They can be quite harsh on the skin if you press too hard, so go gently. Rinse them after use, and allow them to dry naturally. Simply sweep over your body when you're in the shower or bath.
• Your ordinary facecloth or sponge can also double up as an exfoliator. Lather up with plenty of soap or shower gel, and massage over damp skin before rinsing away with clear water.
• Copy what health spas do, and keep a large tub of natural sea salt by the shower. Scoop up a handful when you get in, and massage over your skin. Rinse away thoroughly afterwards.
• You can also make your own body scrub at home by mixing sea salt with body oil or olive oil. Allow the mixture to soak into your skin for a few minutes in order to allow the edges of the salt crystals to dissolve before massaging in, then rinsing away.
• Body brushes are useful. The best way to use them is on dry skin before you get in the bath or shower, as this is very good for loosening dead skin cells. You can also use them in the water, lathering them up with soap or gel.

Perfecting your exfoliation technique

Whichever method you use, the best thing to do is concentrate on problem areas such as upper arms, thighs, bottom heels and elbows. Also sweep over the rest of your body. Go gently on delicate areas of skin, such as the inner arms, stomach and inner thighs. Work in large strokes, in the direction of your heart.
• Oilier skin types will benefit from exfoliation two or three times a week, while once a week is enough for others.
• Never exfoliate broken, inflamed or acne-prone skins.
• After exfoliating, always apply body lotion to seal moisture into the fresh new skin you've exposed.

BEAUTY TIP

For speedy super-soft skin, you should massage your body with oil before climbing into the bath or shower. Then proceed as usual with your preferred exfoliating method.

HAIR REMOVAL

These are the main removal methods for superfluous hair. Each method has advantages and disadvantages, and these have been outlined here:

Shaving

Using a razorblade, shaving works by cutting the hair at the skin surface. It is most effective for legs and underarms.
Pros: Cheap, quick and painless.
Cons: Regrowth (stubble) appears very quickly, usually within a couple of days and you can get razor burn.

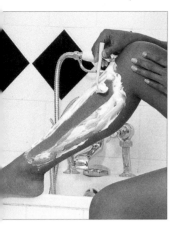

Left For many women, shaving is the no-fuss option for silky smooth legs.

SHAVING TIPS

• Use with a moisturizing shave foam or gel for a close shave. Moisturize afterwards to soothe your skin.

• A closer shave means you will have to shave your legs less frequently.

• Let the shaving cream get to work and soften the hair for a few moments before using your razor.

Tweezing

This rather time-consuming method involves plucking out hairs one at a time so it is most effective for small areas such as eyebrows, or for removing the odd stray hair missed by waxing.

Pros: Good control for shaping.

Cons: Can be painful and may make skin slightly reddened for a short while afterwards. You also need to remember to check the area regularly in a mirror to see that you don't need to re-tweeze. The more often you do it the less it hurts.

TWEEZER TIP

Before you begin, hold a warm facecloth over the area of skin you are going to work on. This will dampen and soften the skin, and open the pores, making tweezing easier and less painful. Or you could try pressing an ice cube over the area to numb the skin first if you find it really painful.

Waxing

This method uproots the hair from below the skin's surface. Either wax is smoothed on to the skin and removed with strips, or pre-prepared wax strips are used. This form of hair removal can be safely used on any part of the body.

Pros: The results last for 2–6 weeks.

Cons: This method can be painful, but the more often you do it the less it hurts. There is also the risk of sore, red and blotchy legs and of ingrowing hairs. Hair has to be left to grow until it is long enough to wax effectively, so you have to put up with regrowth to give the hairs time to grow back sufficiently. If the hair is too short, it won't come out, or it will be removed patchily.

WAXING TIPS

• After waxing the bikini area, apply an antibacterial cream to prevent infection or a rash.

• Wear loose clothing after waxing.

• Never wax a sore area.

Depilatory creams

These creams contain chemicals that weaken the hair at the skin's surface, so hair can be wiped away. Apply, leave for 5–10 minutes, then rinse away (check the packet for instructions). You can use a depilatory cream anywhere, especially as some companies produce different formulations for specific areas. Do a patch test 24 hours before use to make sure it won't cause irritation or an allergy.

Pros: It is cheap, and the results last a bit longer than a razor – up to a week.

Cons: Can be messy and takes time. The smell of some products can be off-putting although most formulations have improved.

Bleaching

This is not technically hair removal, but it's a good way to make hair less noticeable. A hydrogen peroxide solution is used to lighten the hair. Bleaching is best for the arms, upper lip and face.

Pros: Results last between 2 and 6 weeks, and there's no regrowth.

Cons: Not suitable for coarse hair.

BLEACHING TIP

It is a good idea to carry out a patch test on your skin before using to ensure you don't react badly to the product's bleaching agents.

Sugaring

This works in a similar way to waxing, but uses a paste made from sugar, lemon and water.

Pros: Has the same benefits as waxing and can be used anywhere on the body.

Cons: Can be fairly painful and there is a risk of ingrowing hairs.

Laser hair removal

A special implement exposes the hair follicle to pulses of laser light, destroying it. This method is best for small areas and only works on dark, coarse hairs. Make sure you go to a qualified practitioner as their skill and experience are important factors in the procedure's effectiveness.

Pros: A permanent solution.

Cons: Expensive, and can be uncomfortable – it feels like elastic bands snapping against your skin. You may find that you are more sensitive just before or during your period.

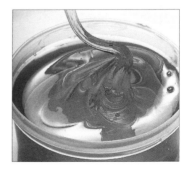

Above Sugaring – the sweeter way of removing superfluous hair.

BEATING CELLULITE

It's not just plumper, older women who suffer from 'orange-peel skin' on their thighs, hips, bottom and even tummy – many slim, young women suffer too. Sadly, there is no miracle cure for cellulite, but there are some practical things you can do to minimize its appearance.

Experts disagree about what causes cellulite. It seems likely that it's an accumulation of fat, fluid and toxins trapped in the hardened network of elastin and collagen fibres in the deeper levels of your skin. This causes the dimpled effect and feel of cellulite areas. These areas also tend to feel cold to the touch because the flow of blood is constricted and the lymphatic system, which is responsible for eliminating toxins, can't work properly. This can worsen the problem and make the cellulite feel puffy and spongy.

TESTING FOR CELLULITE

Try squeezing the skin of your upper thigh between your thumb and index finger. If the flesh feels lumpy and looks bumpy, you have cellulite. Further clues may be that these areas look whiter and feel colder than elsewhere on your legs.

COMMON CAUSES

Cellulite can be caused and/or aggravated by the following:
• A poor diet is full of toxins and puts the body under great strain to get rid of vast quantities of waste. Also, an unhealthy low-fibre, high-fat diet means that the body's digestive system can't work effectively to expel toxins from the body.
• Stress and lack of exercise make your body sluggish and can slow down blood circulation and the lymphatic system.
• Hereditary factors – if your mother has cellulite, you may have it, too.
• Hormones, such as the contraceptive pill or hormone replacement therapy, may contribute.

TACKLING CELLULITE

There are dozens of products around designed to deal with cellulite, but it is debatable how effective they really are.

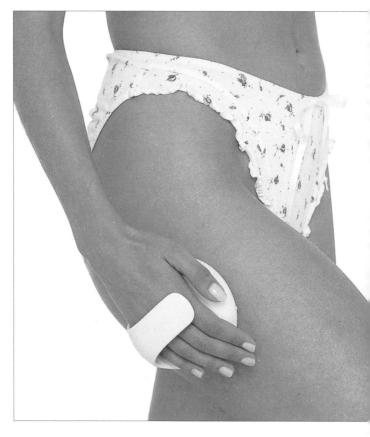

To actually tackle the problem effectively you should attempt to follow a three-pronged approach, combining:
• Circulation-boosting tactics
• Diet
• Exercise

BOOST YOUR CIRCULATION

Here are several ways to boost your circulation and your lymphatic system. Whichever one you choose, aim to follow it for at least 5 minutes a day.
• Use a soft body brush on damp or dry skin. Brush the skin in long sweeping movements over the affected area, working in the direction of the heart.

Above Pep up your circulation and lymphatic system to help beat that cellulite

• Use a massage glove or rough sisal mitt in the same way as you would a body brush.
• Use a cellulite cream. These usually contain natural ingredients such as horse chestnut, ivy and caffeine to boost your circulation. However, you can make them doubly effective by massaging them thoroughly into the skin with your fingertips. Some cellulite creams even come with their own plastic or rubber hand-held mitts to help boost the circulation.

ANTI-CELLULITE DIET

To cleanse your body you need to follow a healthy low-fat, high-fibre diet, such as the one outlined in this three-week weight-loss programme.

Eat at least seven servings of fresh fruit and vegetables every day, trying to make sure you include a good range of different types and colours and eating as many raw or steamed as you can to preserve the nutrient content.

Cut down on the amount of fat you eat. For instance, grill (broil) rather than fry foods, and cut off visible fat from meat. For many foods you buy, look out for a low-fat alternative.

Water cleanses your system and flushes toxins from cells, so drink at least 2 litres (quarts) of fluid daily.

Change from caffeine-laden tea and coffee to herbal teas and decaffeinated coffee. Sip pure fruit juices diluted with water (to reduce the amount of sugar and calories in the drink) rather than high-sugar carbonated drinks.

Steer clear of alcohol as much as possible as it adversely affects your liver – your body's main de-toxifier. Having a hangover will also make it harder to exercise and will make you crave sugary, fatty foods instead of healthy fresh ones.

Drink a glass of hot water containing a slice of a fresh lemon when you get up in the morning – it's a wonderful way to detoxify your body.

Avoid eating processed snacks between meals – eat a piece of fruit, raw vegetables or rice cakes instead.

STEP UP YOUR EXERCISE

Exercise will boost your sluggish circulation and lymphatic system, and encourage your body to get rid of the toxins causing your cellulite. Do a regular aerobic workout, exercising for 20–40 minutes, three to five times a week, and choose from these: brisk walking, swimming, cycling, tennis, aerobic classes or running. (It is always wise to consult your doctor before embarking on a new form of exercise.)

tone it up

You can also try these exercises to increase circulation, firm up your legs and give them a better shape. Carried out daily, they will help you win the cellulite battle.

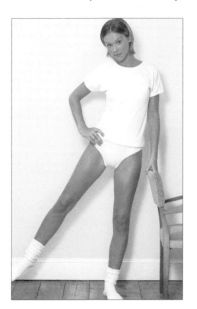

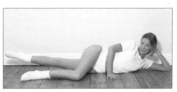

INNER THIGH TONER Lie on your side on the floor, supporting your head with your arm. With your top leg resting on the floor in front, raise the lower leg off the floor as far as you can without straining, then lower it. Repeat 10 times, then turn over and work the other leg.

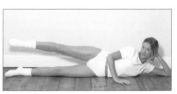

OUTER THIGH TONER Lie on your side, supporting your head with your hand. Bend your lower leg behind you and tilt your hips forwards. Place your other hand on the floor in front of you for balance. Slowly lift your upper leg, then bring it down to touch the lower one. Repeat six times, then work the other side.

HIP TONER Stand sideways with your hand resting on a chair, your knees slightly bent and your shoulders relaxed. Slowly raise your right leg out to the side, keeping your body and raised foot facing forwards. Slowly lower your leg, then repeat this movement 10 times. Turn round and repeat with the other leg.

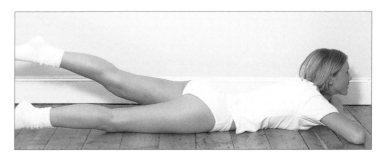

BOTTOM TONER Lie on your front with your hands on top of one another, resting your chin on them if you wish. Raise one leg about 13cm/5in off the floor and hold for a count of 10. Bring your leg back to the floor, and repeat 15–20 times with each leg.

NATURAL BATHING TREATS

Enjoyed in the evening, a body-temperature bath helps the body to relax, absorb the healing benefits of oils and can pave the way for a good night's sleep. Baths also help to ease aching muscles after working out and are a good opportunity to exfoliate your skin or use a face mask.

Although you may be tempted to have a steaming hot bath, a short soak in body-temperature water is more effective at helping you unwind. In addition, bathing in water that is too hot can cause thread veins and may make you feel unwell.

HOME SPA
To make bathing a real indulgence you can create your own aromatic bath products. Lavender, chamomile, clary sage, neroli and rose all have a relaxing, soporific effect.

Add 5–10 drops of your chosen oil blend to your bath, then sink in and relax. Inhaling the aromas will soothe your mind, and the oils will also have a beneficial effect on your skin and body.

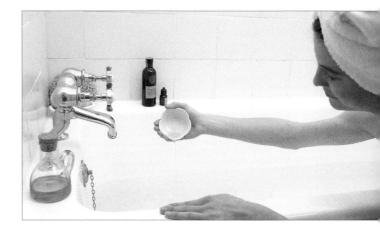

Above Essential oils evaporate very quickly in hot water so the oils will be much more effective if you pour them into body-temperature water just before you climb in.

orange and grapefruit bath oil
At the end of the day, a scented bath is a therapeutic treat. Choose the oils depending on whether you want to be relaxed or invigorated. An orange and grapefruit bath will gently refresh you. Add one teaspoon once you have run the bath, otherwise the oils will evaporate before you get in.

INGREDIENTS
• 45ml/3 tbsp sweet almond oil
• 5 drops grapefruit oil
• 5 drops orange oil

Pour the oils into a bottle and shake them together so that they are well combined before you add 5ml/1 tsp to the bathwater.

goodnight bath salts
Chamomile is a recognized sedative; for these bath salts it has been combined with sweet marjoram, which is another effective treatment for insomnia.

INGREDIENTS
• 450g/1lb/2¼ cups coarse sea salt
• 10 drops chamomile essential oil
• 10 drops sweet marjoram essential oil
• 1–3 drops green food colouring (optional)

Combine all the ingredients and pour into a glass storage jar with a close-fitting lid. Just before bedtime, light a scented candle, add a handful of the salts to your bath, immerse yourself in the warm water and relax.

herbal bath mix
All the ingredients are available to buy or they can be grown in a garden or window box. They are associated with purification and cleansing.

INGREDIENTS
• 7 basil leaves
• 3 bay leaves
• 3 sprigs oregano
• 1 sprig tarragon
• square of cotton muslin (cheesecloth)
• 10ml/2 tsp organic oats
• a pinch rock or sea salt
• thread to tie up muslin

Pile the herbs in the centre of the muslin square, then sprinkle the oats on top. Top with the salt, pick up the corners of the muslin and tie with thread. Hang from the tap so that the water runs through it.

BATHTIME BLENDS
Mix two or three essential oils in a base of sweet almond oil or jojoba oil. These quantities are for a 50ml/¼ cup bottle of base oil. Add 20 drops of the mixed oil to the bathwater. Alternatively, you can mix the oils with an equal quantity of milk or honey because this will help to disperse them in the water. These ingredients also have soothing and softening properties.

• Anti-stress mix: 10 drops each marjoram, lavender and sandalwood.
• Invigorating mix: 5 drops rosemary, 5 drops camphor, 20 drops peppermint.
• Healing mix for colds and flu: 10 drops each eucalyptus, thyme and lavender.
• Soothing arthritis: 30 drops eucalyptus.

MOISTURIZE YOUR BODY

Slick on a body moisturizer every time you have had a shower or bath to create a wonderfully silky body. There are countless different commercially produced gels, creams, mousses and oils on the market, but you can also create your own special moisturizing blend using the recipes given here.

Just as you choose a moisturizer for your face with care, you should opt for the best formulation that is suited to the skin type in your body. These are the most commonly used formulations:

Gels are the lightest formulation and are perfect for very hot days or oilier skin types.

Lotions and oils are good for most skin types, and are easy to apply.

Creams give better results for those with dry skins, especially on dry areas.

MAKE THE MOST OF MOISTURIZER

Apply moisturizer using firm strokes to boost your circulation.

Apply the moisturizer straight on to clean, damp skin – after a bath or shower is the ideal time. This helps seal extra moisture into the upper layers of your skin, making it softer than ever.

Soften cracked feet by rubbing them with rich body lotion, pulling on a pair of cotton socks and heading for bed.

SMELLING SCENT-SATIONAL

Opt for a scented body lotion as a treat – they can often be longer-lasting than the eau de parfums they are based upon. Alternatively, use them as part of 'fragrance layering'. This simply means taking advantage of the various scent formulations available. Start with a scented bath oil and soap, move on to the matching body lotion and powder, and leave the house wearing the fragrance itself sprayed on to pulse points. However, be careful you don't clash fragrances. Choose unscented products if you're also wearing perfume, unless you're going to be wearing a matching scented body lotion. You don't want cheaper products to compete with perfume.

• Concentrate on rubbing moisturizer into particularly dry areas such as heels, knees and elbows. The calves are also very prone to dryness because there aren't many oil glands present there.

• If you don't have time to apply moisturizer after your bath, simply add a few drops of body oil to the water. When you step out of the bath, your skin will be coated with a fine film of nourishing oil. Always remember to rinse the bath well afterwards to prevent you from slipping the next time you climb into the bath.

• Your breasts don't have any supportive muscle from the nipple to the collarbone and skin is fine here. Firming creams won't work miracles, but can maintain the elasticity and suppleness of this delicate area. Regular application of body lotion can have similar effects.

HOME-MADE LOTIONS

For pure pampering pleasure nothing beats a tailor-made beauty preparation, and you can choose the ingredients specially to suit your own skincare needs. Mixing oils or adding your favourite essential oil to a ready-made unscented cream is easy to do and very rewarding and is also cheaper than buying comparable commercial products.

geranium body lotion

This is a spicy, fragrant lotion. Geranium oil is derived from a relative of the scented geranium leaf and the fragrance is pleasantly sharp and aromatic.

INGREDIENTS

• 175ml/6fl oz unscented body lotion
• 15 drops geranium essential oil

Add the geranium oil to the body lotion, mix well and pour into a bottle with a tight lid.

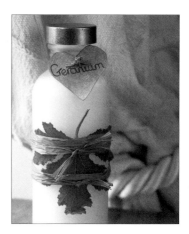

Above It is a good idea to label and date home-made lotion. It should keep for a month or so if it is stored in a sealed bottle in a cool place, but will not keep indefinitely.

coconut and orangeflower lotion

This creamy preparation is soothing and nourishing for dry skin. Wheatgerm oil is rich in vitamin E, an antioxidant that protects skin cells against premature aging.

INGREDIENTS

• 50g/2oz coconut oil
• 60ml/4 tbsp sunflower oil
• 10ml/2 tsp wheatgerm oil
• 10 drops orangeflower essence or 5 drops neroli essential oil

1 Melt the coconut oil in a heatproof bowl over a pan of gently simmering water. Stir in the sunflower and wheatgerm oils. Leave the mixture to cool, then add the fragrance and pour into a jar, seal and label with the name of the mixture and the date.

2 The lotion will solidify after several hours. For the best results warm the cream in your hands briefly before applying it liberally to dry areas of skin.

NATURAL BODY TREATS

Many more of us are waking up to the benefits of aromatherapy and natural beauty products these days, and for very good reasons. Natural therapies are wonderful to use, easily available and can give immediate results, but there are a few people who cannot use them, so check first.

Aromatherapy uses essential oils, which are the distilled essences of herbs, plants, flowers and trees. These oils smell wonderful and are a pleasure to use. It's this smell that usually attracts people to them for treating a variety of physical and mental conditions, from skin infections to stress, as well as for their beautifying powers.

TIPS FOR USING ESSENTIAL OILS

• Essential oils are natural products but their effects can be powerful, so they must be used with care.
• If you don't want to buy individual essential oils, buy them ready-blended, or treat yourself to bath and body products that contain them.
• Some oils are thought to carry some risk during pregnancy. For this reason, consult a qualified aromatherapist for advice before using them if you are pregnant or trying for a baby and want to use essential oils.
• Don't treat medical conditions with essential oils – consult your doctor.
• Essential oils can be expensive, but a little goes a long way.
• Do not apply essential oils undiluted as they're too concentrated in this form and can result in inflammation. The only exception is lavender, which can be used directly on the skin for insect bites and stings. Otherwise, mix essential oils with a carrier oil.
• Don't take essential oils internally. Essential oils are about 50 to 100 times more powerful than the plant from which they were extracted and can be harmful if consumed.
• Don't apply oils to areas of broken, inflamed or recently scarred skin.

• Whichever method of aromatherapy you use, shut the door to the room.
• For immediate results add 4 drops of your chosen oil to a bowl of hot water, lean over it and cover your head with a towel. Inhale for about 5 minutes.
• Place a few drops of your favourite oil on a tissue, so you can inhale it whenever you like. Eucalyptus is great for blocked sinuses or if you have a cold. Alternatively, sprinkle a few drops of chamomile or lavender on your pillow to help you sleep.
• If you have sensitive skin, carry out a patch test. Apply diluted oil to a small patch of skin and leave it for a few hours to make sure you do not have an adverse reaction to it.

AROMATHERAPY MASSAGE
Mix 3–4 drops of essential oil into 10ml/2 tsp of a neutral carrier oil such as sweet almond oil, and use to massage your body – or ask someone else to massage you.

SOAPS AND SCRUBS
In addition to adding essential oils to the bathwater, you can create lovely soaps and scrubs that you apply directly to your skin while bathing or taking a shower.

lavender and olive oil soap
Use a good-quality pure olive oil soap to make this soap. Enrich it with other oils and scent it with lavender to produce a rejuvenating cleanser.

INGREDIENTS
• 175g/6oz good-quality olive oil soap
• 25ml/1½ tbsp coconut oil
• 25ml/1½ tbsp almond oil
• 30ml/2 tbsp ground almonds
• 10 drops lavender essential oil
• lavender buds for decorating

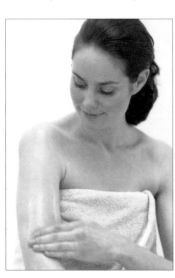

Above For a soothing and moisturizing massage on a problem area, mix 15ml/1 tbsp almond oil with a suitable essential oil and massage gently. Breathe deeply as you rub to maximize the therapeutic effect.

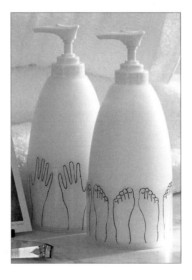

Above Keep home-made moisturizing lotions, such as these ones for the hands and feet, in pump-action bottles, since these make dispensing the cream easier and will mean you will use them more frequently.

grate the soap and place in a double boiler. Leave the soap to soften over a low heat. When soft, add the other ingredients and mix. Press the mixture into oiled moulds and leave to set overnight. Unmould, then decorate by pressing the top of each block of soap into a shallow tray of picked lavender buds.

citrus body scrub

Orange peel is mixed with the ground sunflower seeds, oatmeal and sea salt in this scrub, helping to remove dead skin cells and stimulate the blood supply to the skin, leaving it feeling toned and smooth.

INGREDIENTS

- 45ml/3 tbsp freshly ground
  sunflower seeds
- 45ml/3 tbsp medium oatmeal
- 45ml/3 tbsp flaked sea salt
- 45ml/3 tbsp finely grated
  orange peel
- 3 drops grapefruit essential oil
- almond oil

Mix together all the ingredients except the almond oil and store in a sealed glass jar. Using just a little at a time, mix with some almond oil to make a thick paste, then rub over damp skin.

applying a body scrub

For smoother, softer skin, mix the scrub with water or oil to make a paste.

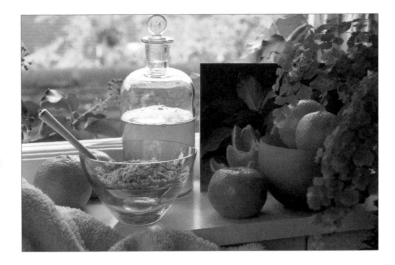

HAND AND FOOT CREAM

These creams are made by adding essential oils to an unscented cream, which means that you can adapt the recipe to suit you. Look out for a lanolin-rich cream or one that includes cocoa butter, as hands and feet benefit from richer formulations. Although most creams and lotions are best stored in glass or ceramic containers, in this case it is practical to keep the lotion in a pump-action plastic bottle, which makes it much easier to use.

Above The combination of aromatic orange peel and refreshing grapefruit oil in this body scrub gives it a stimulating, clean scent.

tea tree foot cream

Tea tree is one of the best essential oils to add to a foot cream. It has healing, antiseptic properties and an effective fungicidal action.

INGREDIENTS

- 120ml/4fl oz unscented cream
- 15 drops tea tree essential oil
- bowl and spoon for mixing
- pump-action plastic bottle
- funnel

Blend the oils into the unscented cream and pour into the plastic bottle through a funnel.

healing hand cream

In this nourishing cream the chamomile soothes, the geranium helps heal cuts and the lemon softens the skin.

INGREDIENTS

- 120ml/4fl oz unscented hand cream
- 10 drops chamomile essential oil
- 5 drops geranium essential oil
- 5 drops lemon essential oil
- bowl and spoon for mixing
- pump-action plastic bottle
- funnel

Blend the oils into the hand cream and pour into the plastic bottle through a funnel.

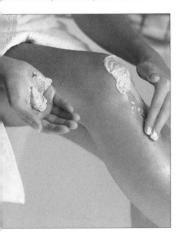

1 Work the scrub into damp skin using firm pressure, paying particular attention to areas of dry skin such as the elbows and knees.

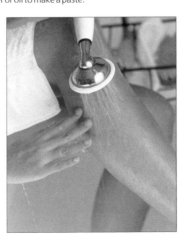

2 Use a dry flannel to remove most of the scrub and then gently rinse the rest away with warm water.

FOOT PAMPERING

Setting aside time for a regular treatment will help you to care for your feet and keep them healthy all year round. A pamper session once a month will greatly improve their appearance, and will also soften the skin and help boost the circulation.

You'll need at least an hour to do the treatment on this page properly – or you can really indulge yourself and take two hours for the session. Use this as a time to relax – you will find that focusing on your feet is a great way to forget about day-to-day worries.

foot pamper routine

This routine uses the luxury foot scrub (opposite). If you don't have time to make this, buy one from a store that includes essential oils so that you can benefit from their soothing properties, which are especially desirable if you have been pounding a treadmill or swimming, which can dry out skin. You also need foaming bath or foot gel, a foot bowl, one large towel and two smaller ones, two bags that are large enough to slip your feet into, a pumice stone and pedicure tools.

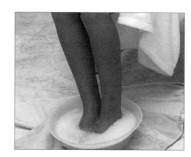

1 Half fill a large bowl with warm water. Place the bowl on a large towel on the floor. Add a little foaming gel, and perhaps a couple of drops of essential oil that have been diluted first in a carrier oil. Swish the water around with your hand to create bubbles and to release the aroma of the essential oil. Put both feet into the water, then sit back and relax as you soak them for 5 minutes. Remove your feet from the bowl and rub on the floor towel to remove most of the water.

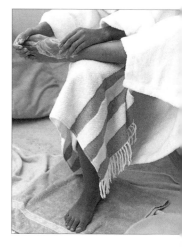

2 Put a towel on your right knee and rest the left foot on top. Massage the foot scrub all over the sole, paying extra attention to any rough skin, and rub into the cuticles. Place your foot in a plastic bag and secure.

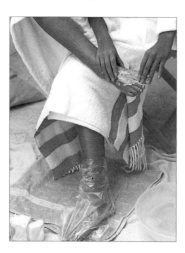

3 Repeat on the right foot. Wait 10 minutes, then remove the bag from the left foot, sliding it down the foot to remove the foot scrub. Do the same for the right foot. Dip both feet into the water. This will have cooled down, so it will stimulate the circulation.

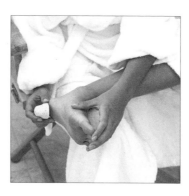

4 Remove your feet from the bowl. Place your left foot on the right knee. Take the pumice stone and rub over the sole. Use firm pressure on the heel and ball, and light pressure on the arch. Now rub the pumice all over the top of the foot, using light pressure. This helps to improve the skin texture and bring nutrient-rich blood to the surface, which will help improve the appearance. Repeat on the left foot.

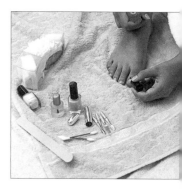

5 Trim the nails straight across, then smooth the edges with an emery board. Use a cotton bud (swab) to apply cuticle remover, wait a few minutes, then gently push the cuticle back with a hoof stick. Soak the feet again, then carefully clean under the nail. Dry the feet, then apply base coat, polish and top coat, using cotton wool (cotton) to separate the toes and allowing each layer to dry before applying the next.

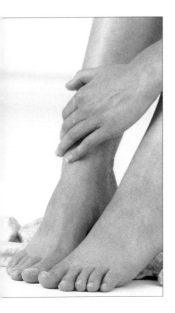

Left Soft, manicured feet are a real asset, especially during the warmer summer months when they are likely to be on show.

INGREDIENTS
• 5ml/1 tsp each almond oil, jojoba oil and glycerine – to nourish and soften the skin
• 5ml/1 tsp each Fullers earth and rock salt – to soften and cleanse
• 10ml/2 tsp foaming foot or bath wash – to cleanse the skin and soften the cuticles
• 3 drops essential oil – for aromatic feel-good factor. Choose whichever oil you like best, or you could use a blend: mandarin and geranium, or lavender and lemon are relaxing, cleansing combinations

In a small clean bottle, mix the foaming wash, essential oil and glycerine. Shake and set aside while you prepare the other ingredients. Put the Fullers earth and rock salt into a medium-sized dish and mix together. Mix in the almond and jojoba oils. Add the glycerine mixture to the bowl, and mix all the ingredients together with a metal spoon. You should now have a runny paste.

luxury foot scrub

The following recipe is an excellent cleanser and softener for the feet. It can be used whenever you feel they need a boost. For the best results, though, set aside enough time for a long pamper session to enable the moisturizer to really sink in.

lemon verbena and lavender foot bath

This refreshing foot bath will soothe tired feet after an aerobic session.

INGREDIENTS
• 15g/½oz dried lemon verbena
• 30ml/2 tbsp dried lavender
• 5 drops lavender essential oil
• 30ml/2 tbsp cider vinegar

Put the lemon verbena and lavender into a basin and pour in enough hot water to cover the feet. When it has cooled add the lavender oil and cider vinegar. Sit down and immerse your feet in the bath for 15 minutes. Dry your feet thoroughly afterwards.

CARING FOR YOUR FEET

A pedicure will help to keep your feet attractive and healthy. You will need a few special items, but because they will last a long time they are definitely a worthwhile investment.

• **Nail-polish remover:** It's a good idea to choose a conditioning one.
• **Cotton wool (cotton):** Ideal for removing nail polish and also useful for separating toes while you paint them.
• **Nail brush or orange stick (tip covered with cotton wool):** Useful for cleaning under the nail.
• **Hoof stick or cotton buds (swabs):** Vital for pushing back the cuticles.
• **Toenail clippers:** These are often easier to use than scissors.
• **Emery board:** Toenails are harder than fingernails so you'll need a strong one.
• **Cuticle remover:** Invaluable for softening and loosening the cuticle.
• **Nail polish and a clear top coat:** Great for sealing and preventing chipping.

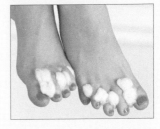

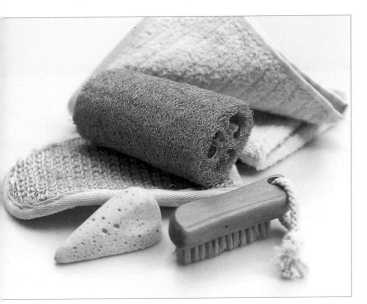

Above After soaking your feet in a footbath for 10 minutes, use a loofah or nail brush to scrub and cleanse, then use a pumice on the dead skin all over the soles of the feet. Pat them dry, then give your feet a quick massage using neroli and lemon essential oils well diluted in almond oil.

BEAUTIFUL NAILS

Regular care and a little manual labour is all it takes to have nails that you will want to show off, rather than ones you want to hide away. If you are going out or have a special occasion to attend, you may want to try adding some colour or going for a chic French manicure.

Our hands go through a lot and deserve a little special care and attention. Try to wear gloves when washing up or doing housework, or when the weather is cold.

HEALTHY NAILS

There's no point slicking your nails with colour if they're not in good condition to start with. Following this advice will ensure that they're ultra-tough.

Filing know-how

Keep your nails slightly square or oval – not pointed – to prevent them from breaking. Filing low into the corners and sides can weaken nails. File gently in one long stroke, from the side to the centre of the nail. The classic length that suits most hands and doesn't get in the way is just over the fingertip.

Condition-plus

Smooth your nails every evening with a nourishing oil or conditioning cream. This helps seal moisture into your nails to prevent flaking and splitting. A tiny drop of olive oil is a great cheap and natural alternative.

Cuticle care

Go carefully with tough or overgrown cuticles. Most manicurists are against cutting them with scissors, as this can lead to infection. Instead, soak your nails in warm soapy water to soften the cuticles. Then smooth them with a little cuticle softening cream or gel, before gently pushing them back with a manicure hoof stick or clean cotton bud (swab). You can then gently scrub away the flakes of dead skin that are still clinging to the nail bed.

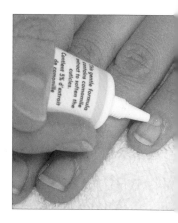

Above Soften cuticles with a cream or gel before pushing them back.

CUTICLE COLOUR CODING

• If you have long, elegant fingers you can carry off any shade, including the dramatic deep reds, russets and burgundies. Short nails look best with pale or beige-toned polish.
• Pale colours also suit broad nails, but you can make them look narrower by leaving a little space at the sides of each nail unpainted.
• If you love barely-there shades for the daytime, but prefer something more exotic at night, try a pale pearlized polish – the shimmer will be caught by the evening light.
• If you find strong colours too bold on your fingers, try painting your toenails instead. A glimpse of colour in open-toed shoes or on bare feet can look sophisticated. You can create a great look by mixing a little dark red and black nail polish before applying.
• Coral polish and pearlized formulations work very well against a tanned skin.

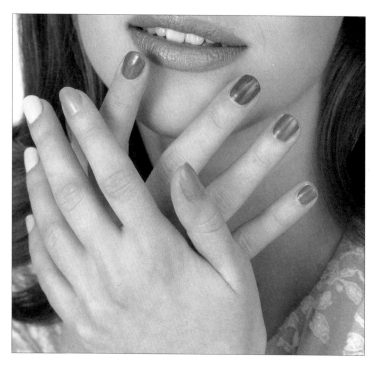

Left There is a huge range of different nail polish colours and finishes to explore in order to find shades that suit you.

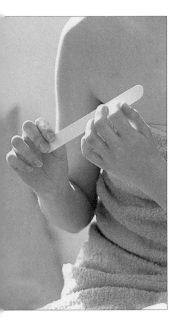

Left Fingernails should be filed regularly. To minimize breakage, file them straight across with a soft emery board.

French manicure

This is a popular look because it makes all lengths of nail look clean and healthy. It combines white tips with a pink polish over the entire nail. It is suitable for all occasions, from an ultra-natural to a glamorous look. It does take a little practice at first, but it's worth persevering. There are also special kits that contain all you need to get it right.

BEAUTIFUL NAIL TIP

The key to perfecting the French manicure, or indeed any manicure, is to be very patient! It is important that you wait for each coat to dry thoroughly before applying the next one. If you rush the stages and apply the coats too quickly, the manicure will not be perfect because you are sure to end up with smudges and a rather messy finish. Wait until you can dedicate about 30 minutes to the process before beginning – perhaps once the children are in bed!

OP 10 NAIL TIPS

Avoid using acetone nail polish emovers, as these can strip your nails f essential moisture. Choose the onditioning variety instead.

Apply hand cream every time you vash your hands. The oils in the cream vill seal moisture into your skin.

The most common cause of soft nails , exposure to water, so wear rubber loves when doing the dishes.

If you have weak nails, try painting our base coat and nail polish under the ips to give them extra strength.

Dry wet nails in an instant by lunging them into ice-cold water.

To repair a split nail, tear a little paper rom a teabag and glue it over the tear vith nail glue. Once it's dry, buff until mooth then apply polish on top.

If you're planning to do some ardening or messy work, drag your ails over a bar of soap first.

Clean ink and stains from your ingertips by using a toothbrush and oothpaste on the affected areas.

Don't file your nails immediately after bath, as this is when they're at their veakest and most likely to split.

0 Use a cotton bud with a pointed end o clean under your nails – it's gentler han scrubbing with a nail brush.

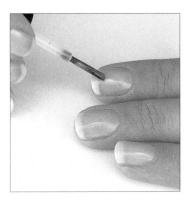

1 Apply a clear base coat to protect your nails and help to prevent chipping.

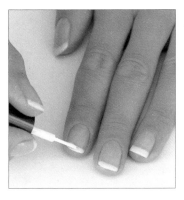

2 Apply two thin coats of white polish to the tips of your nails. Try to apply it in one long stroke, working from one side of your nail to the other.

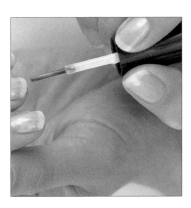

3 Allow the white polish to dry completely, then apply a coat of pink polish over the entire nail. If you like a very natural finish, apply just one coat of pink polish; if you prefer a bolder effect, apply two coats.

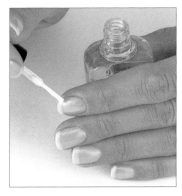

4 Apply a clear top coat over the entire nail for added protection.

FACE PAMPERING

For deep-down cleansing and a definite improvement in skin tone, try these simple recipes and techniques to get a salon-perfect complexion. They cost a fraction of a professional facial, take very little time and can be done in the privacy of your own home at a time that suits you.

'Cleanse, tone and moisturize' should be your mantra for everyday healthy skin, and you need to do this morning and night. To give skin a boost, you should also try to include a facial once a week, especially if you are exercising, as sweat can make you prone to spots.

SKIN TONIC RECIPE

This flower skin tonic is suitable for normal skin, and can be applied to soothe and freshen the skin.

INGREDIENTS
• 75ml/5 tbsp orangeflower water
• 25ml/1½ tbsp rosewater

Pour the ingredients into a glass bottle and shake to mix. Apply to skin with a cotton wool (cotton) pad.

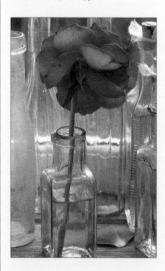

Above If you make your own rosewater any fragrant roses are suitable for this recipe, as long as they have not been sprayed with pesticide, but pink or red ones smell best.

freshening facial

Facial skin is delicate and needs regular cleansing to keep the pores dirt-free so the skin can breathe.

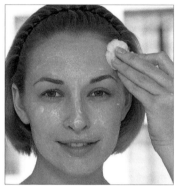

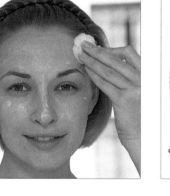

1 Smooth your skin with cleansing cream. Leave on for 1–2 minutes to give it time to dissolve grime, oil and stale make-up. Then gently smooth away with a cotton wool (cotton) ball.

2 Dampen your skin with warm water. Gently massage with a blob of facial scrub, taking care to avoid the delicate eye area. This will loosen dead surface skin cells, and leave your skin softer and smoother. It will also prepare your complexion for the beneficial treatments to come. Rinse away with splashes of warm water.

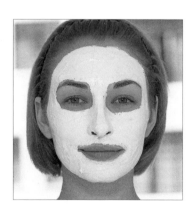

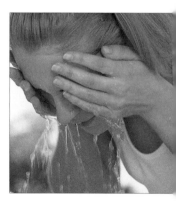

4 Smooth on a face mask. Use a clay-based one if you have oily skin or a moisturizing type if you have dry or normal skin. Leave the mask on your skin for 5 minutes, or for as long as specified on the product.

5 Rinse away the face mask with warm water. Once all the mask is removed, finish off with a few splashes of cool water to close your pores and freshen your skin, then pat dry gently with a towel.

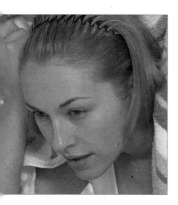

Fill a bowl or washbasin with boiling water. Lean over it, capturing the steam with towel placed over your head. Let the steam warm and soften your skin for 5 minutes. you have blackheads, try to remove them ently with tissue-covered fingers after this eatment. Do not do this if you suffer from ensitive skin or are prone to broken veins.

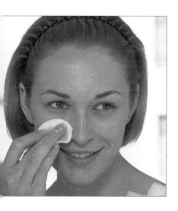

Soak a cotton wool pad with a skin toner ation or a home-made tonic (such as the ne in the box opposite), and smooth over ly areas of the face, such as the nose, chin nd forehead.

face massage

Dot your skin with moisturizer and smooth in. Following your facial, continue the pampering by taking the opportunity to massage your skin, as this encourages a brighter complexion and can help to reduce puffiness.

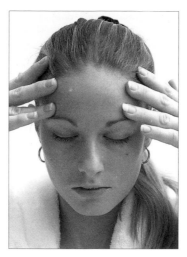

1 Starting in the centre of your forehead, make small circular motions with your fingertips and work slowly out towards the temples. Repeat three times.

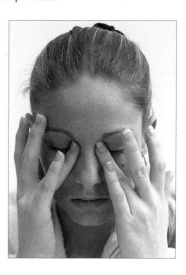

2 Use your ring fingers to apply gentle pressure to the area where the eye socket meets your nose. Hold for 5 seconds. Repeat at least three times.

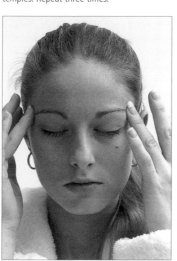

3 Move your fingers outwards along the brow bone from the top of your nose. Repeat five times. The skin around the eyes is the most delicate on the face and the first to show signs of stress, so it is important that you treat this area very gently. Use your middle fingers, as these are the weakest and will apply the softest pressure.

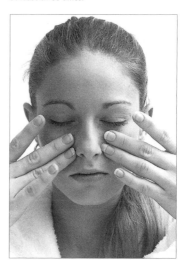

4 Starting either side of your nose, move your fingers outwards using circular motions along the cheekbone to the jaw. Pay particular attention to the jaw area. Repeat five times. Finally, gently smooth your undereye area with a soothing eye cream to reduce fine lines and wrinkles, and make the skin ultra-soft.

CARE FOR EYES

The fine, delicate skin around your eyes is the first to show the signs of ageing. However, don't be tempted to deal with the problem by slapping on heavy oils and moisturizers because they are usually too heavy for the skin in the eye area. They can also block tear ducts, causing puffiness.

The delicate skin around your eyes needs particularly special care because it is significantly thinner than the skin on the rest of your face, and this means that it is less able to hold in moisture. There are also fewer oil glands in this area, making it particularly susceptible to dryness, and also meaning that there is no fatty layer underneath to act as a shock absorber. Consequently this area of skin quickly loses its suppleness and elasticity.

CHOOSING AN EYE TREATMENT

There is a huge range of products to choose from, and it is important to find the right one for you. Gel-based ones are suitable for young or oily skins, and are refreshing to use. However, most women find light eye creams and balms more effective.

Use a tiny amount of the eye treatment, as it's better to apply it regularly in small quantities than apply lots occasionally. Apply with your middle finger, as this is the weakest

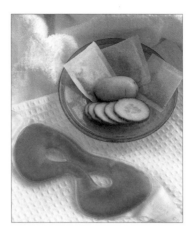

Above There is a range of remedies for eyes, from special pads to home-made therapies. Experiment to find out which works for you.

one and won't stretch the delicate skin. This will help keep your skin more supple and prevent premature wrinkling in this area.

PREVENTING PUFFY EYES

This is one of the most common beauty problems. These ideas can help:
• Gently tap your skin with your ring finger when you're applying eye cream to encourage the excess fluid to drain away.
• Store creams in the refrigerator, as the coldness will also help to reduce any puffiness.
• Place thin strips of potato underneath your eyes to reduce swelling. The starch in the potato seems to tighten the skin.
• Fill a small bowl with iced water or ice-cold milk. Soak two cotton wool (cotton) pads and lie down with the pads over your eyes. Replace the pads as soon as they become warm. Continue for 15 minutes. This treatment reduces puffiness and brightens the whites of your eyes.

COOLING CUCUMBER

This is a quick and simple treatment. Place a slice of cucumber over each eye, then just lie back and relax for 15 minutes. Cucumber will gently tone and soothe the skin around the eyes.

HERBAL EYEPADS

A compress over your eyes will refresh, reduce puffiness and relieve itchiness.

fennel decoction

Make a decoction by boiling 10ml/2 tsp fennel seeds in 300ml/½ pint/1¼ cups purified water for 30 minutes. Strain and cool, then use to soak cotton wool pads.

teabag treatments

Use a teabag to make tea then apply to the eyes when cool. Chamomile tea is good for tired eyes. The tannin in Indian tea is an astringent and will firm the skin.

rosewater

Soak cotton wool pads in an infusion of rose petals and purified water.

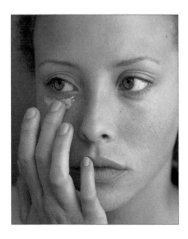

Above The skin around the eyes is soft and delicate so it is important to apply moisturizer to this area very gently.

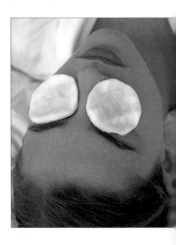

Above Whichever eye treatment you decide to use, it is vital that you take time to lie down and relax for at least 10 minutes.

GOODNIGHT CREAMS

Going to bed with night cream on your face can benefit your skin while you are sleeping. The main difference between night creams and ordinary daily moisturizers is that most night creams have special added ingredients such as vitamins and anti-ageing components.

They can also be thicker and more intensive than creams you apply during the day because you won't need to apply make-up on top of them. Your skin's cell renewal is more active during the night, and night creams are designed to make the most of these hours. Using a night cream gives your skin the chance to repair the daily wear and tear caused by pollution, sweating, make-up and ultra-violet light.

WHO NEEDS NIGHT CREAMS?

While very young skins do not generally require the extra nourishing properties of night creams, most women will benefit from using one regularly. Dry and very dry skins will respond particularly well to this treatment. Remember that you don't have to choose very rich formulations, as there

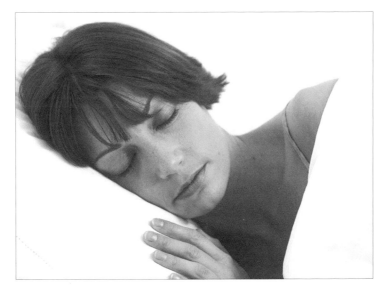

Below Dab a little night cream in your palm, then rub your hands together. The heat will liquefy the cream so that it is more easily absorbed as you massage it into your skin.

are lighter alternatives that contain the same special ingredients. Choose which formulation you use carefully on the basis of how dry your skin is – it is important that your skin shouldn't feel overloaded.

Above Applying night cream before you go to bed means waking up to a softer, smoother complexion. If you apply cream to slightly damp skin this can boost its performance, as it seals in extra moisture. Let it sink in before placing your face on the pillow.

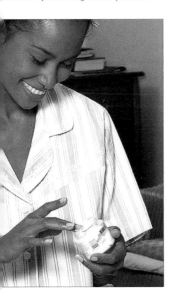

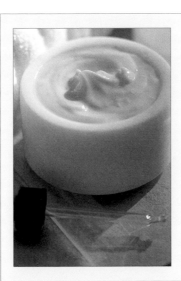

NOURISHING NIGHT CREAM

As we get older, our skin becomes drier and more in need of regular care. Jasmine and rose oils help to rehydrate the skin, while frankincense helps reduce wrinkles and restore tone to slack muscles.

INGREDIENTS
- 50g/2oz jar of unperfumed base cream with a close-fitting lid
- 3 drops of rose essential oil
- 2 drops of frankincense essential oil
- 1 drop of jasmine essential oil

Add the oils to the cream and mix everything together well. Apply a little of the cream just before going to bed.

SPECIAL SKIN TREATMENTS

As well as basic moisturizers, there is a vast range of special treatments, serums and gels that have been carefully formulated to treat specific problems available in stores. The selection can be a bit baffling, so here is a brief low-down on what products are and what they do.

Knowledge is power, so arm yourself with the facts before spending a fortune on facial products. Special skin treatments come in all shapes and sizes, and in various different formulations, outlined below, so there is something for everyone.

SERUMS AND GELS

These have an ultraviolet formulation, a non-greasy texture and a high concentration of active ingredients. They're not usually designed to be used on their own, except on oily skins. They're generally applied under a moisturizer to enhance its benefits and boost the anti-ageing process.

SKIN FIRMERS

You can lift your skin instantly with creams that are designed to tighten, firm and smooth. They work by forming an ultra-fine film on the skin, which tightens your complexion and reduces the appearance of fine lines. The effects last for a few hours, and make-up can

easily be applied on top. These products are a wonderful treat for a special night out or when you're feeling particularly tired.

SKIN ENERGIZERS

These creams contain special ingredients designed to accelerate the natural production and repair of skin cells. As well as producing a fresher, younger-looking skin, they are also thought to help combat the signs of ageing.

AMPULE TREATMENTS

These concentrated active ingredients are contained in sealed glass phials or ampules, to ensure that they're fresh. Typical extracts include herbs, wheatgerm, vitamins and collagen – used for their intensive and fast-acting results. Vitamin E or evening primrose oil is another great skin saver. Break open a capsule and smooth the oil on to your face using your fingers for a fast skin treat.

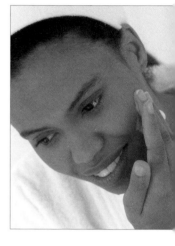

Above Choose a cream that contains specialized ingredients to improve your skin.

Liposomes creams

These are tiny spheres in the cream which carry special ingredients into the skin. Their shells break down as they're absorbed into your skin, releasing the active ingredients.

AHA KNOW-HOW

Alpha-hydroxy acids, also commonly known as fruit acids, are found in natural products. These include citric acid from citrus fruit, lactic acid from sour milk, tartaric acid from wine, and malic acid from apples and other fruits. Incorporated in small amounts, AHAs are often a key ingredient in specialized skincare products.

They work by breaking down the protein bonds that hold together the dead cells on the surface of your skin. They then lift them away to reveal brighter, plumper cells underneath. This gentle process cleans and clears blocked pores, improves your skin tone and softens the look of fine lines. Basically, they're the ideal solution to most minor skincare problems. You should see results within a couple of weeks, although many women report an improvement after only a few days.

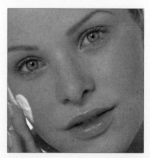

Without even realizing it, women have used AHAs for centuries and have reaped the benefits for their skins. For example, Cleopatra is said to have bathed in sour asses' milk, and ladies of the French court applied wine to their faces to keep their skin smooth and blemish-free – both these ancient beauty aids contain AHAs.

AHA products are best used under your everyday moisturizer as a treatment cream. You should avoid applying them to the delicate eye and lip areas. If you have sensitive skin, you may find they're not suitable for you. Some women experience a slight tingling sensation as the product gets to work. The great news is that AHA products are now becoming more affordable, and not just the preserve of more expensive skincare companies. Many mid-market companies are including the benefits of AHAs in their products, so anyone can give their skin the treatment it deserves.

10 WAYS TO BEAT WRINKLES

ine lines and wrinkles aren't inevitable. In fact, skin experts believe that most skin damage can be revented with some special care. Here are the 10 main points to bear in mind, no matter what our age, to ensure your skin stays as young-looking as possible.

SUN PROTECTION
he single biggest cause of skin ageing sunlight. Use a sunscreen every day ecause the aging effects of the sun re as prevalent in the winter months as the summer ones. This will help prevent our skin from aging prematurely, and ill guard against burning.

STOP SMOKING
igarette smoke speeds up the ageing rocess as it strips your skin of oxygen nd slows down the regeneration of ew cells. It can give the skin a grey, uggish look, and cause fine lines round the mouth.

DEEP CLEANSE
is essential to ensure your skin is ear of dead skin cells, dirt and make-p to give it a youthful, fresh glow. on't use harsh products – a creamy eanser removed with cotton wool otton) is effective for most women. your skin is very dry, massage with oily cleanser. Leave on your skin or a few minutes, then rinse away the xcess with warm water.

DEEP MOISTURIZE
s well as using a daily moisturizer, you an also boost your skin's water levels eekly. Either use a nourishing face ask, or apply a thick layer of your sual moisturizer or night cream. Vhichever you choose, leave on the kin for 5–10 minutes, then remove he excess with tissues. Apply to damp kin for greater effect.

BOOST THE CIRCULATION
uy a gentle facial scrub or exfoliater, nd use once a week to keep the urface of your skin soft and smooth. his increases the blood-flow to the top yers of skin, and encourages cell

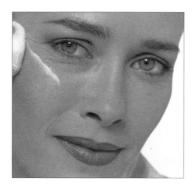

Above Whatever you are applying to your skin, use gentle strokes and an upwards motion.

renewal. You can get the same effect by lathering a facial wash on your skin using a clean shaving brush.

6 DISGUISE LINES
Existing lines can be minimized to the naked eye by opting for the latest light-reflecting foundations, concealers and powders. These contain luminescent particles to bounce light away from your skin, making lines less noticeable and giving your skin a wonderful luminosity.

7 PAMPER REGULARLY
As well as daily skincare, remember to treat your skin from time to time with special treatments such as facials, serums and anti-ageing creams.

8 BE WEATHER VAIN
Extremes of cold and hot weather can strip your skin of essential moisture, leaving it dry and more prone to damage. Central heating can have the same effect. For this reason, ensure you moisturize regularly, changing your products according to the seasons. For instance, in the winter you may need a more oily product, which will

keep the cold out and won't freeze on the skin's surface. In hot weather, lighter formulations are more comfortable on the skin, and you can boost their activity by using a few drops of special treatment serum underneath.

9 BE GENTLE
Be careful not to drag at your skin when applying skincare products or make-up. The skin around your eyes is particularly likely to show signs of ageing. A heavy touch can cause the skin to stretch. So, always use a light touch, and take your strokes upwards, rather than drag the skin down. Also, avoid any products that make your skin itch, sting or feel sensitive. If any product causes this sort of reaction, stop using it at once and switch to a gentler formulation.

10 BE GENTLE
Skincare products are not the only things that can benefit skin; in fact, many make-up products now contain UV filters and skin-nourishing ingredients to treat your skin as well as superficially improve its appearance. So investigate the latest products – it's well worth making use of them.

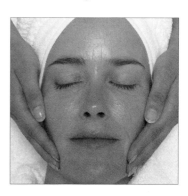

Above Relax and enjoy a beneficial facial!

20 SKINCARE QUESTIONS ANSWERED

Everybody is unique, but some skin problems seem to occur time and again and can cause concern and frustration. To beat those skin blues, here are quick and simple remedies, and sound advice, for a range of common skincare problems, both for the face and the body.

1 NIGHT WATCH

Q *'My skin needs night cream, but I seem to lose most of it on my pillow.'*
A Try placing the cream in a teaspoon, and heating it gently over a low heat on the stove until it is just warm, before applying. It sounds strange, but it really works!

2 POLISHED PERFECTION

Q *'I spend a fortune on skincare, but resent paying for exfoliators. Are there alternatives?'*
A Yes. After washing your skin, gently massage with a soft facecloth or natural sponge to ease away the dead surface skin cells. If you have dry skin, massage cream cleanser on to damp skin, then rub over the top with your flannel. Rinse, then apply moisturizer in the normal way. It is essential to wash the facecloth after every couple of uses, and to hang it up to dry in between to prevent the build-up of bacteria.

3 LIP TRICKS

Q *'How can I stop my lips getting so chapped and flaky in winter?'*
A This three-step action plan will help:
• Massage dry lips with petroleum jelly. Leave for a couple of minutes to soften the skin, then gently rub your lips with

a warm, damp facecloth. As the petroleum jelly is removed, the flakes of skin will come with it!
• Smooth your lips morning and night with a lip balm.
• Use a moisturizing lipstick to prevent lips drying out during the daytime.

4 RED NOSE DAY

Q *'How can I cover my red nose?'*
A Try smoothing a little green foundation or concealer over the red area before applying foundation and powder. The green works by cancelling out the redness.

5 WINTER SUN

Q *'Is it true that you should still wear a sunscreen in winter?'*
A Yes. Exposure to sunlight is thought to be the main cause of wrinkling, and the ultraviolet A rays that are responsible for this process are around all year, so choose a moisturizer that contains sunscreens.

6 LIGHTEN UP

Q *'My skin feels as though it needs a richer cream in the winter months, but I find most of them too heavy'*
A A heavier moisturizer doesn't necessarily mean it's more effective, so choose one that feels right for you. Help seal moisture into your skin by spritzing your face with water before applying it. Also, choose a nourishing foundation or tinted moisturizer to ensure your skin stays smooth and soft all day long.

7 WATER FACTOR

Q *'I like the feeling of water on my face, but I find using soap and water too drying. Should I switch to a cream cleanser instead?'*

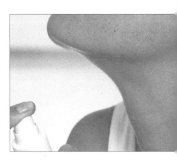

Above Boost the moisture in your skin with refreshing spritz.

A For dry skin, it's generally better to use a creamy cleanser – applied with your fingertips and removed with cotton wool (cotton) or soft tissues. This prevents too much moisture from being lost from the skin's surface. Normal and oily skins should be fine with water but use a facial wash or wash-off cleanser that is formulated to be non-drying, while still cleaning your skin.

8 AGE SPOTS

Q *'I've noticed 'liver spots' on the back of my hands. How are they caused – and how can I get rid of them?'*
A Many people find these light-to-dark brown patches on the back of their hands as they grow older. They can also appear on the forehead and temples. They're caused by an uneven production of the melanin tanning pigment in the skin. This can be caused by excess sun exposure, or merely highlighted by it.
You can use a cream containing hydroquinone, which penetrates the skin tissue to 'dissolve' the melanin. In six to eight weeks, your skin should be back to normal. However, you must use a safe level of hydroquinone – the recommended amount in a cream is

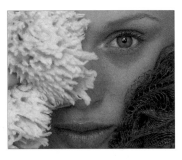

Above The soft touch of a natural sponge is a cheap and effective alternative to a facial.

wo per cent. Using a sunscreen on a aily basis can prevent these patches rom appearing again.

SENSITIVE SKIN
Q *'Why does my skin feel more ensitive in winter than in summer?'*
A Eighty per cent of women claim to ave sensitive skin – which tingles, tches and is prone to dryness. It can e aggravated by harsh winter winds nd cold, because this breaks down he natural protective oily layer. Moisturizing regularly with a hypo-llergenic cream formulated for ensitive skin should help.

0 PREGNANT PAUSE
Q *'I'm pregnant and have patches of darker colour on my face, particularly under my eyes and around my mouth. What is this?'*
A This is called chloasma, or 'the mask of pregnancy'. It's triggered by a hange in hormones, and is made more bvious by sunbathing. Cover up in the un and use sunblock to stop patches ecoming denser. It usually fades vithin a few months of having your aby. Chloasma can also be triggered y birth-control pills, but disappears nce you stop taking them.

1 ON THE SPOT
Q *'I suffer from oily skin, but find lemish creams too drying. What an you suggest?'*
A Choose an antibacterial cream to kill ff the cause of your blemishes while oothing the skin around them.

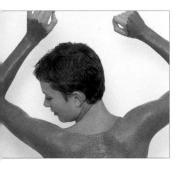

Above Back to basics with a clay body mask.

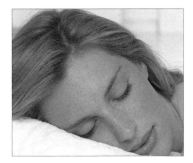

Above Don't forget your beauty sleep.

12 TREATMENT SPRAYS
Q *'I find body lotions too hot and sticky to wear after bathing. What else can I try?'*
A There are body treatment sprays, combining moisturizer, toner and fragrance. Your skin will be lightly moisturized and smell fantastic.

13 THE THROAT VOTE
Q *'The skin on my neck looks grey and dull. Are there any special treats to use?'*
A Necks show the signs of ageing, mainly because they lack sebaceous glands. Dull grey skin benefits from regular exfoliation and boost softness by smoothing on moisturizer.

14 BEAUTIFUL BACK
Q *'What can I do for pimples on my back?'*
A Backs are hard to reach, so they're prone to break-outs. Try exfoliating daily with a loofah or back brush. For stubborn pimples, try a clay mask to draw out deep impurities.

15 MOLE WATCH
Q *'How do I keep an eye on moles on my skin?'*
A Moles are clumps of clustered pigment cells, usually darker than freckles. All changes in existing moles should be checked by your doctor. Any that cause concern will be removed and sent off for analysis. You should also check moles yourself once a month. Try the following A.B.C.D. code: check for A (asymmetry); B (border irregularity); C (colour change); D (change in diameter).

16 SHADOW SENSE
Q *'What's best for shadows under my eyes?'*
A Dark shadows can have a variety of causes, including fatigue, anaemia, lack of fresh air and poor digestion. They can also be hereditary. If in doubt, consult your doctor. Take steps to cut out causes by getting a good night's sleep and keeping to a low-fat, high-fibre diet. Try bathing the eyes with pads soaked in ice-cold water for 15 minutes, to lessen the shadow effect temporarily. Or cover with concealer.

17 BROWN BABY
Q *'Is there a way to prolong a tan?'*
A Your skin is dried by sunbathing, and so sheds old cells more quickly. Prolong colour by applying lots of body lotion. Use while your skin is damp to make it extra effective. Apply a little fake tan every few days to keep your colour topped up. Better still, protect your skin by using fake tan all the time.

18 STICKY SITUATION
Q *'I exercise a lot, and find body odour a problem. How can I prevent it?'*
A Sweating is your body's natural cooling device. Sweat itself has no odour, but smells when it comes into contact with bacteria on the skin. So, opt for an antiperspirant deodorant and wear natural fibres next to your skin.

19 MASSAGE MAGIC
Q *'Can I give myself a facial massage?'*
A Yes – see the massage on page 127.

20 STRETCH MARKS
Q *'Can I get rid of the stretch marks on my stomach, breasts and thighs?'*
A Stretch marks are a sign of your skin's inability to cope with the rapid expansion of flesh underneath. The collagen and elastin fibres underneath actually tear with the strain. They usually appear in times of rapid weight gain. There's nothing you can do once you've got them, except wait until they start to fade. However, moisturizing well can help guard against them.

MAKE-UP BASICS

Being considered beautiful today no longer means conforming to one accepted ideal. The modern approach to beauty places the emphasis firmly on the individual and her own particular needs, aspirations and lifestyle. For although every woman is concerned to some extent about how she looks, everyone is very different and has varying expectations.

No matter what you look like, make-up can be used to enhance your features. Applied with a sensitive touch it should create a subtle emphasis, rather than a mask disguising the features.

Many women are wary of cosmetics because they are not sure which colours suit them or which make-up methods and textures are the most flattering. Good make-up hinges on experience: you learn what suits you by trial and error. Nobody wants to waste money on a lipstick that turns out to be the wrong colour when you try it at home; but it's easy to get stuck in a rut – so be brave and experiment a little.

PRODUCT KNOW-HOW
No two women are alike. When we're buying a pair of jeans, we don't just pick the same size, colour and pair as our sister, because we have different

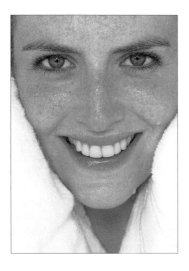

Above Take a close look at your face while you are washing or getting ready for bed. Which features would you like to enhance and which would you like to play down?

requirements. Make-up is the same. We need to choose carefully from the vast array of products and formulations around to create a look that's made-to-measure for our own complexions and features. Buying the most expensive product on the shelves is no guarantee of success, as it may not be the most suitable for your colouring or skin type.

The next few pages will take you through the myriad bottles, compacts and colours, and show you how to find the ones that work best for you, and how to apply them.

TAILOR-MADE MAKE-UP
The perfect make-up for you will be effortless once you choose the correct shades for your skin tone and hair colour. It'll also work wonderfully, because you'll still look like you, only better! Checking your hair colour is easy – whether it's natural or comes out of a bottle. Deciding whether your skin is 'warm' or 'cool' seems slightly more difficult – however, there is an easy way to check. Simply look in a mirror and hold a piece of gold and a piece of silver in front of your face. These can just as easily be pieces of foil or costume jewellery as the real thing. The right metal will bring a healthy glow to your skin, whereas the wrong will make it look grey. If gold suits your skin, then it's 'warm' toned. If silver suits it, it's 'cool' toned. A further clue is how well you tan in the sun – cool skin tones tend to colour less easily.

HOW TO REASSESS YOUR IMAGE
Take a careful look at your make-up bag or drawer. How old are the cosmetics? Six months, a year or more? Now study your face when you are wearing your usual make-up, and ask

yourself what exactly your make-up does for you: does it widen or narrow your eyes or mouth, enhance the shape of your face, make you look younger or older? If it does not produce the effect you require and your cosmetics are more than a year old, it is time for a complete change. However, you should bear these points in mind before you rush out to the nearest store:

Your age: Make-up that suited you when you were 25 is not going to look right 10 years down the line. Changes in skin tone and texture, as well as in hair colour, require different make-up shades, properties and textures: the right make-up can take years off your face.

Your face shape and skin tone: Make-up can improve face shape by illusion; it can also improve skin tone and texture.

Your eye colour and size: Deftly applied make-up can make small eyes look bigger, blue eyes look bluer and round eyes look longer; can your current make-up do this for you?

Your hair colour: Make-up should complement the shade of your hair; if your hair is jet black and your skin is pale, deep red lipstick and black eye make-up (mascara and kohl) look stunning. If you are blonde, earthy tones look best (the bright colours can be a bit brassy). If you have brown or black hair, you will have almost limitless colour freedom.

Your lifestyle: Make make-up easy; there is no point choosing make-up that requires a great deal of time to apply properly if you have a busy lifestyle. If you have a baby or small children you are likely to look tired, but a good under-eye concealer and a subtle blusher can work wonders.

MAKE-UP TOOLS

Even the most expensive make-up in the world won't look particularly great if it's applied carelessly and using your fingertips. For a professional finish you need the right tools. This means investing in a set of decent brushes and applicators and taking good care of them. As with many pieces of equipment, buy the best you can afford and do your research.

There is a mind-boggling range of make-up tools available on the market, and the price can vary tremendously. Before you go shopping, it is worth taking the time to consider exactly what you need, depending on what make-up you use, and doing a little research to see which would be best for your budget and your lifestyle. For instance it is better to invest in a compact for a handbag rather keeping an expensive brush and loose powder rattling around in a bag.

MAKE-UP SPONGE
Have a wedge-shaped one, so you can use the finer edges to help blend in foundation round your nose and jawline, and the flatter edges for the cheeks, forehead and chin. However, if you prefer not to use a synthetic sponge try the small, natural ones instead. Remember to use it damp, not dry.

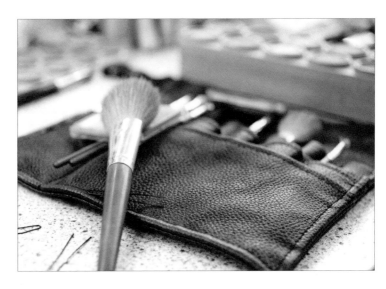

Above You can buy smart sets of make-up brushes. Although the initial outlay may seem considerable, the sets are usually more cost-effective than buying individual brushes.

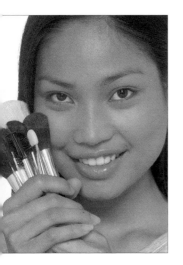

Above Armed with a selection of good-quality tools you will be able to apply make-up better and produce really stunning results with little effort.

POWDER BRUSH
Get used to using a powder brush each time you put make-up on. To prevent a caked or clogged finish to your face powder, use a large, soft brush to dust away any excess.

BLUSHER BRUSH
Use to add a pretty glow to your skin with a light dusting of powder blusher. A blusher brush is smaller than a powder brush to make it easier to control, but you could use a powder brush if you don't want to buy both types.

EYESHADOW BRUSH
Smooth on any shade of eyeshadow with this small, soft brush. It may be worth having one for dark colours and one for light shades.

EYESHADOW SPONGE
A sponge applicator is ideal for applying a sweep of pale eyeshadow that doesn't need much blending, or for applying highlighter to your brow bones.

ALL-IN-ONE EYELASH BRUSH/COMB
Great for combing through your lashes between coats of mascara for a clump-free finish. Flip the comb over and use the brush side to sweep your eyebrows into shape, or soften pencilled-in brows.

LIP BRUSH
Create a perfect outline and then use it to fill in the shape with your lipstick.

EYEBROW TWEEZERS
It is essential to have a good pair of slanted tweezers for regularly tidying up the eyebrows.

EYELASH CURLERS
Once used, curlers soon become a beauty essential! Curlier eyelashes make a huge difference to the way your lashes look and help open up the eyes.

FOUNDATIONS AND CONCEALERS

Many women avoid foundation because they're scared of an unnatural, mask-like effect. In fact, finding the right product for your skin is simpler than you might think. Concealers are a fast and effective way to disguise blemishes, shadows, scars and red veins, so your skin looks perfect.

There are two keys to success when it comes to using foundation: the first is to pick the right formulation, and the second is to choose the perfect shade for your skin.

FIND YOUR FORMULATION

Long gone are the days when you could only buy heavy pancake foundation. Now you can choose from many formulations, so you can get the best coverage for your particular skin type. Here are the products on offer, and who they're best for.

Tinted moisturizers

These are a cross between a moisturizer and a foundation, as they'll soothe your skin while giving a little coverage. They're ideal for young or clear skins. They're also great in the summer, when you want a sheer effect or to even out a fading tan. Unlike other foundations, you can blend tinted moisturizers on with your fingertips.

Liquid foundations

These are the most popular and versatile of all foundation types,

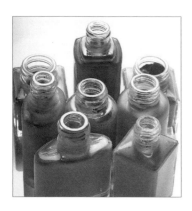

Above It is well worth spending time to find the right foundation colour for you.

because they smooth on easily and offer natural-looking coverage. They suit all but the driest skins. If you have oily skin or suffer from occasional spot break-outs, look for an oil-free liquid foundation, to cover the affected areas without aggravating them.

Cream foundations

These are thick, rich and moisturizing, making them ideal for dry or mature skins. As they have a fairly heavy texture, make sure you blend them well with a damp cosmetic sponge.

Mousse foundations

Again these are quite moisturizing and ideal for drier skins. The best way to apply the product is to dab a little on to the back of your hand, then dot it on to your skin with a sponge.

Compact foundations

These are all-in-one formulations, which already contain powder. They come in a compact, usually with their own sponge for application. However, they actually give a lighter finish than you'd expect. They're great on all but dry skin types.

Stick foundations

These are the original foundation. They have a heavy texture, and so are best confined for use on badly blemished or scarred skin. Dot a little foundation directly on to the affected area, then blend gently with a damp sponge.

SHADE SELECTION

Once you've chosen the ideal formulation for you, you're ready to choose the perfect matching shade for your skin. At last cosmetic companies have woken up to the fact that not everyone has an 'American

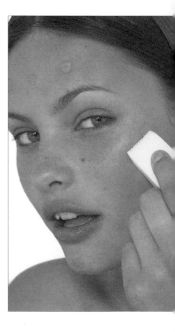

Above Blend, blend, blend for a professional finish. And don't forget to give all angles of your face a final check in the mirror to make sure you haven't got any unnatural lines where your foundation finishes.

tan' complexion! Now, there is a good selection of foundation shades from a pink-toned English rose to a yellow-hued, olive skin, as well as from the palest skin to the darkest one.

Here are some tried-and-tested methods for choosing the perfect one for your skin tone:
• Ensure you're in natural daylight when trying out foundation colours, so you can see exactly how your skin will look once you leave the store or make-up counter.
• Select a couple of shades to try that look as though they'll match your skin.
• Don't try foundation on your hand or on your wrist – they're a different colour to your face.

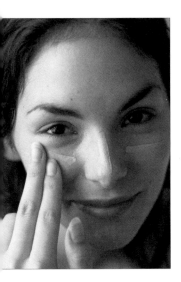

• Stroke a little colour on to your jawline to ensure you get a tone that will blend with your neck as well as your face. The shade that seems to 'disappear' into your skin is the right one for you.

APPLICATION KNOW-HOW
Apply foundation to freshly moisturized skin to ensure you have a perfect base on which to work.
• Use a cosmetic sponge to apply most types of foundation – using your fingertips can result in an uneven, greasy finish.
• Apply foundation in dots, then blend each one with your sponge.
• Dampen the sponge first of all, then squeeze out the excess moisture – this will prevent the sponge from soaking up too much costly foundation.
• Check for tell-tale 'tidemarks' on your jawline, nose, forehead and chin.

HIGH-PERFORMANCE FOUNDATION
Companies these days have made great improvements to their foundations. Here are some benefits to look out for:
• Many companies have added sunscreens to their foundations, so they'll protect you from the ageing effects of the sun while you wear them. Look out for the words UV Protection and Sun Protection Factor (SPF) numbers on the tube or bottle.

• Look for 'light-diffusing' foundations, which are great for older skins. They contain hundreds of tiny light-reflective particles that bounce light away from your skin – making fine lines, wrinkles and blemishes less noticeable.

CORRECT COLOUR
You can wear a colour-corrective foundation underneath your normal-hued foundation to alter your skin-tone. They can seem quite strange at first glance but are, in fact, highly effective at toning down a high colour or boosting the colour of your complexion. Use them sparingly at first until you feel confident that you have achieved an effective, but subtle, result.
• Green foundation cools down rosiness and is great for those who blush easily.
• Lavender foundation will brighten up a sallow complexion, and is great for when you're feeling tired.
• Apricot foundation will give a subtle glow to dull skin, and is a great beauty booster in the winter.
• White foundation gives a wonderful glow to all complexions, and is perfect for a special night out.

WHAT ARE CONCEALERS
Concealers are concentrated foundation with a high pigment content, giving complete coverage to problem areas. Make-up artists argue as to whether concealer should be applied before or after foundation. Applying it after foundation is often best, as it's applied to specific areas which would be disturbed when the foundation was applied. If you're after a light effect, apply concealer to clean skin, then apply powder or all-in-one foundation/powder on top.

Stick concealers
These are easy to apply as you can simply stroke them straight on to the skin. Some have quite a thick consistency, so it's worth trying samples before buying.

Cream concealers
These usually come in a tube, with a sponge-tipped applicator. The coverage isn't as thick as the stick type, but the finished effect is natural.

Liquid concealers
Again, these come in a tube. Just squeeze a tiny amount on to your finger and smooth over the affected area. Look for the cream-to-powder formulations, which slick on like a cream and dry to a velvety powder finish.

TAKING COVER
Here's how to conceal all your beauty problems effectively.

Spots and blemishes
The ideal solution is to use a medicated stick concealer as this contains ingredients to deal with the pimple or blemish as well as cover it. Only apply the concealer on the pimple or blemish, as it can be quite drying, and then smooth away the edges with a clean cotton bud (swab). Applying concealer all around the area will make the spot more noticeable.

Under-eye shadows
Opt for a creamy stick concealer or a liquid one. If you're blending with your fingertips, use your ring finger, as this is the weakest finger and less likely to drag at the delicate skin around your eyes.

Scars
Scars, including old acne or chickenpox marks, can be covered using a concealer but it can be a time-consuming process. Begin by building the indentation up to skin level by dotting on layers of concealer using a fine brush. Take your time and allow each layer to settle into the skin properly.

Red veins
Stick or liquid concealer is ideal for tackling this problem. Apply a layer of concealer over the area with a fine eyeliner brush or clean cotton bud, then feather and soften the edges to blend them in and make them less noticeable.

THE POWER OF POWDER

Face powder is the make-up artist's best friend, as it can make your skin look really wonderful and is very versatile in its uses. It often needs topping up throughout the day to remove shine, so it is worth carrying a small powder compact in your handbag to keep you looking fabulous all day long.

Here are four good reasons for putting on that powder!
• Powder gives a smooth sheen to your skin – with or without foundation.
• It 'sets' your foundation, so it stays put and looks good for longer.
• Powder absorbs oils from your skin, and helps prevent shiny patches appearing as you rush around.
• It helps conceal open pores.
You'll need two types of powder – a loose form at home, and a powder compact for your handbag.

LOOSE POWDER
This gives the best and longest-lasting finish and is the choice of professional make-up artists and models. The most effective way to apply loose powder is to dust it lightly on to your skin using a large, soft powder brush. Then lightly brush over your face again to dust off the excess.

PRESSED POWDER
Compacts containing pressed powder are ideal for carrying in your make-up bag as they're very quick to use and lightweight. Most come with their own

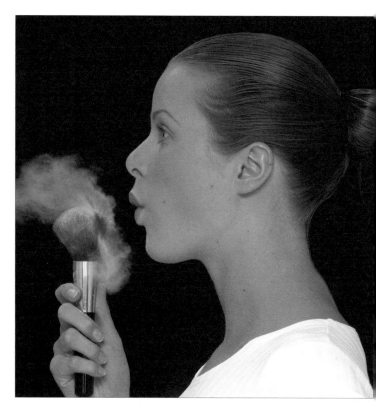

application sponges, but you'll find you get a better result if you apply them with a brush. Look for brushes with retractable heads to carry in your make-up bag.
   If you do use the sponge, use a light touch and wash it regularly, or you'll transfer the oils in your skin on to the powder and get a build-up.

SHADE AWAY
Don't make the mistake of thinking that one shade of powder suits all. Instead, choose one that closely matches your skin-tone for a natural effect. Do this by dusting a little on your jawline, in the same way as you would with foundation.

Above Careful application of the right powder as the final finishing and fixing touch should give your skin a soft, glowing and natural feel.

POWDER TIP
When dusting excess powder away from your skin, use your brush in light, downward strokes to help prevent the powder from getting caught in the fine hairs on your skin. Pay particular attention to the sides of the face and jawline which aren't so easy for you to see. Try not to get powder in your hairline or especially in your eyebrows or lashes, as it can irritate your eyes.

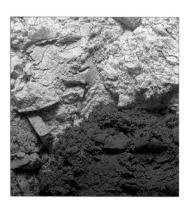

Above Take time to experiment so you choose the shade that best suits your colouring.

BEAUTIFUL BLUSHER

Blusher is an instant way to give your looks a lift. It's old-fashioned to use blusher to sculpt your face, as it looks so unnatural. Instead, it should be applied in the way it was first intended to be used – to recreate a youthful flush on the apples of the cheeks.

Give your complexion a bloom of colour with this indispensable beauty aid. There are two main types, both of which have their merits.

POWDER BLUSHER

This should be applied over the top of your foundation and face powder. To apply powder blusher, dust over the compact with a large soft brush. If you've taken too much on to your brush, tap the handle on the back of your hand to remove the excess. It's better to waste a little blusher than to apply too much as it is hard to tone down! A good guide is to use half as much blusher and twice as much blending as you think you need. You don't want to look like a clown.

Start applying the colour on the fullest parts of your cheeks, directly below the centre of your eyes. Then smile and lightly dust the blusher over your cheekbones and up towards your temples. Blend the colour well towards the hairline, so you avoid harsh edges. This will effectively place colour where you would naturally blush and subtly enhance your cheekbones.

CREAM BLUSHER

Breaking all the traditional beauty rules, cream blusher is applied with your fingertips. It's put on after foundation and before face powder. It drops out of fashion from time to time, but it's never long before it makes a comeback. This is for good reason, as it can give a lovely fresh glow to every skin type.

To apply, dab a few dots of cream blusher over your cheeks, from the plump part up towards your cheekbone. Using your fingertips, blend well. Build up the effect gradually, adding more blusher to create just the look you want. Or, if you prefer, use a foundation wedge to blend in cream blusher.

COLOUR CHOICE

There is a kaleidoscope of blusher shades to choose from. However, as a rule, it's best to opt for a shade that tones well with your skin colouring, and co-ordinates with the rest of your make-up. You can go for lighter or darker shades, depending on the season. As when choosing foundation, check the colour in daylight.

BLUSHER COLOUR GUIDE

Colouring	Choose
Blonde hair, cool skin	Baby pink
Blonde hair, warm skin	Tawny pink
Dark hair, cool skin	Cool rose
Dark hair, warm skin	Rosy brown
Red hair, cool skin	Soft peach
Red hair, warm skin	Warm peach
Dark hair, olive skin	Warm brown
Black hair, dark skin	Terracotta

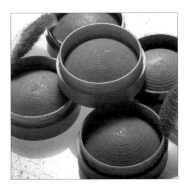

Below Be a blushing beauty with a light touch of powder blusher (left). Or go for more of a glow with cream blusher (right).

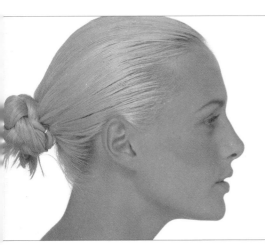
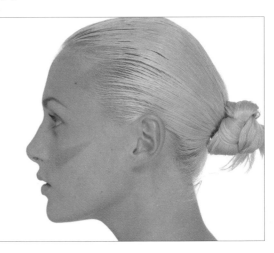

EYE-CATCHING MAKE-UP

Eye make-up is the most popular type of cosmetic, and for good reason. Just the simplest touch of mascara can open up your eyes, while a splash of colour can transform them instantly. Whatever your eye shape and colour, you can take steps to ensure that they always look stunning.

Many women hesitate to experiment with eye make-up because it seems too time-consuming and complicated. The sheer quantity of products on the shelves can make it more intimidating. However, you can create a huge variety of looks – from the simplest to the most extreme – by opening your eyes to the basic techniques.

EYEBROW KNOW-HOW

Many women ignore their eyebrows completely. Or sometimes, which is even worse, they will overpluck them. When it comes to eye make-up, the eyebrows make an important impression. They can provide a balanced look to your face so it's well worth making the effort to master the techniques and seeking professional advice when it comes to reshaping them to get them looking right.

For perfectly groomed brows in an instant, try combing through them with a brush, combing the hairs upwards and outwards. This will also help give you a wide-eyed look. Then lightly slick them with clear gel to hold the shape in place.

LINING UP LINER

Eyeliner can be applied to flatter all eye shapes and sizes. If you have never applied eyeliner before, try this technique. Sit down in front of a mirror in a good light. Take your eyeliner in your hand and rest your elbow on the table to keep your arm and hand steady. You might want to give yourself extra support by resting your little finger on your cheek. Eyeliner should be applied after eyeshadow and before mascara.

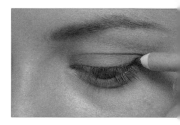

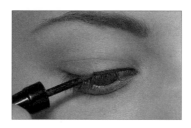

Liquid liners
These have a fluid consistency, and usually come with a brush attached to the cap. To apply, look down into a mirror to prevent smudging. Stay like this for a few seconds after applying to give it time to dry.

Pencil liners
This is the easiest way, and one of the most effective, to add emphasis to your eyes. Using a pencil, draw a soft line, keeping close to your upper lashes, then repeat under your lower lashes.

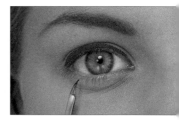

FALSE EYELASHES
These luscious lashes are great for party looks but they can be tricky to apply. The strip lashes can look too

define your eyebrows with powder or pencil colour

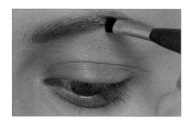

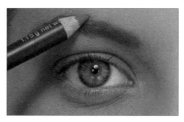

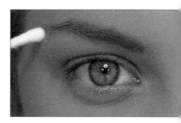

1 To define your brows you can use eyebrow powder or pencil. Apply powder with an eyebrow brush, dusting it through your brows without sweeping it on to the surrounding skin. This gives a natural effect.

2 Alternatively, you could use a well-sharpened pencil to draw on tiny strokes, taking care not to press too hard or the finished effect will be unnatural and could seem odd if this is not your intended look.

3 Soften the lines you've made with the pencil by lightly stroking a cotton bud (swab) through your brows. If you do not like the result, you can remove the powder or pencil using a cotton bud and make-up remover.

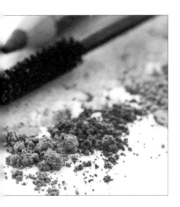

bove Experiment with the wonderful range
f colours of mascara, eye pencils and
yeshadows on offer.

bvious unless you apply them perfectly.
's a better idea to use the individual
ashes on the outer corners of your
yes. Dot the roots with a little glue,
hen use a pair of tweezers to position
hem exactly.

MAGIC MASCARA

Mascara creates a flattering fringe to
our eyes – particularly if your lashes
re fair. Most mascaras are applied
with spiral wands that are quick and
asy to use. Some contain fibres to
dd length and thickness. Opt for a
waterproof variety to withstand tears,
howers and swimming – but
emember you'll need a special eye
make-up remover as it clings more
ercely to your lashes.

EYING UP EYESHADOWS

Choose neutral colours to enhance
your looks subtly, or play with a
kaleidoscope of different shades.
• **Powder eyeshadows:** The most popular
type, these come in pressed cakes of
powder either with a small brush or a
sponge applicator. You can build up
their density. Apply with a damp brush or
sponge for a deep colour.
• **Cream shadows:** These are oil-based
and come in pots or compacts. They're
applied with either a brush or your
fingertips and are a good choice for dry
or older skins that need moisturizing.
• **Stick shadows:** These are wax-based
and smoothed on to eyelids from the
stick. Ensure they have a creamy texture
before you buy, so they won't drag at
your skin.
• **Liquid shadows:** Usually these come in
a slim bottle with a sponge applicator.
Look out for the cream-to-powder ones
that smooth on as a liquid and then
blend to a velvety powder finish.

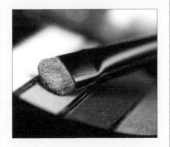

eyeshadow as eyeliner

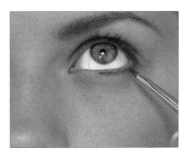

1 Make-up artists often use eyeshadow
to outline the eyes, and it's a trick worth
stealing! It looks very effective because it
gives a soft smoky effect. Use a small, fine
brush to apply shadow under your lower
lashes and to make an impact over the top
of the eyelid, taking care to keep the shadow
close to the eyelashes.

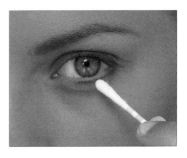

2 To create an even softer effect, simply
sweep over the eyeshadow liner with a
cotton bud, or apply another layer and blend
it in for a stronger effect.

imple steps for creating perfect lashes

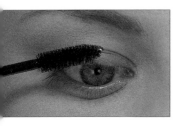

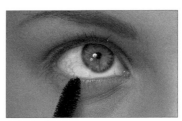

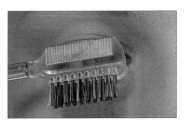

1 Start by applying mascara to your upper
ashes. Brush them downwards to start with,
hen brush them upwards from underneath.
Use a tiny zigzag movement to prevent
mascara from clogging on your lashes.

2 Next, use the tip of the wand to brush your
lower lashes, using a gentle side-to-side
technique. Take care to keep your hand
steady while you are applying the mascara,
and don't blink while the mascara is still wet.

3 Comb through your lashes with an eyelash
comb to remove any excess, and to prevent
clumping. For a more defined effect, repeat
the two previous steps twice more, allowing
each layer to dry before applying the next.

20 MAKE-UP PROBLEMS SOLVED

Whether you've made a mistake and created a wonky line of eyeliner or applied too much blusher, have run out of a vital product or are simply stuck for inspiration, the following problem solvers will give you all the help you need to maximize your beauty potential.

1 POLISH REMOVER HAS RUN OUT

If you want to re-paint your nails, but have run out of remover, try coating one nail at a time with a clear base coat. Leave to dry for a few seconds, then press a tissue over the nail and remove it quickly – the base coat and coloured polish will come off in one quick move.

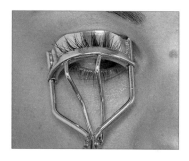

2 POKER-STRAIGHT EYELASHES

A set of eyelash curlers can make a significant difference to the way your eyes look. Gently squeeze your upper lashes between the cushioned pads to curl your lashes beautifully.

3 PATCHY POWDER

If you apply powder with a light touch to freshly moisturized skin, or on top of foundation that is applied with a clean sponge, it should look perfect. If it doesn't, check you're not making the mistake of using the wrong colour powder for your skin. It needs to be matched closely to your natural skin tone, as closely as your foundation. So, try dusting powder on to your skin in natural daylight before buying it, to check you've found the perfect match.

4 YELLOW NAILS

Yellow nails are usually caused by wearing dark-coloured nail polish without using a protective clear base coat, so wear one in future to prevent this from happening. You can also try switching to paler-coloured polishes that contain lower levels of pigment so are less likely to stain your nails.

To cure yellow nails, rub with lemon juice to remove stains, then massage your hands and nails with moisturizer. Try going polish-free one day a week. If your problem recurs, consult your doctor to check that there's no underlying cause.

5 FLAKY MASCARA

This usually means the mascara is too old and the oils that give it a creamy consistency have dried out. This can be made worse by pumping air into the dispenser when replacing the cap. Replace your mascara every few months.

Revive an old mascara by dropping it into a glass of warm water for a few minutes before applying. If mascara flakes on your lashes, the only solution is to remove it and make a clean start.

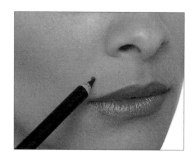

6 A BLEMISH APPEARS

The immediate solution is to transform the blemish into a beauty mark! First, soothe the blemish by dabbing it with a gentle astringent on a clean cotton bud (swab). This will dry out excess oils from the skin and help the beauty mark last longer. To create your beauty mark, dot over the top with an eyebrow pencil – this is better than using an eyeliner pencil as it has a drier texture and so is less likely to melt and smudge. Finally, set your beauty mark in place with a light dusting of loose powder.

7 MELTING LIPSTICK

If you're out and your lipstick is starting to melt, dust over the top with a little loose powder. This will give a slightly drier texture and help the lipstick stay put for longer. Loose powder will also create a matte finish.

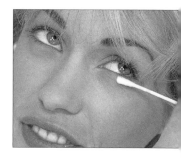

8 SMUDGED EYELINER

Tidy under-eye areas by dipping a cotton bud in eye make-up remover. Whisk it over the problem area to remove smudges, then re-powder. A little loose powder over eyeliner will combat the smudging that occurs as the wax in the pencil melts.

9 RED SKIN

A red skin colour can be toned down by smoothing your skin with a specialized green-tinted foundation. Apply with a light touch to the areas that really need it. The green pigment in the cream has the effect of cancelling out the red in your skin. To avoid a ghostly glow, apply a light coating of your ordinary foundation on top, set with a dusting of loose powder. This tip is also good for covering an angry spot or blemish.

10 FOUNDATION TURNS ORANGE

Mix 5g/1 tsp of bicarbonate of soda (baking soda) into your loose face powder, then dust the powder mixture lightly over your skin before applying your foundation. The bicarbonate of soda will give your skin a slightly acid pH to prevent it from turning orange.

11 BLEEDING LIPSTICK

A lipliner can prevent lipstick from bleeding into the fine lines around your mouth. Trace the lip outline, then apply lip colour with a brush. A drier-textured matte lipstick is less prone to bleed than the moisturizing variety. Also, lightly powder over and around your lips before you start.

12 DISAPPEARING FOUNDATION

If your foundation seems to sink into your skin on hot or damp days, apply it to cool skin. Do this by holding a damp facecloth on to your skin for a few moments, then apply your foundation. Storing foundation in the refrigerator will ensure it's cool when it goes on. Apply the foundation with a damp sponge, not your fingers, as the oils from your skin will leave a streaky finish. Set with a light dusting of loose powder.

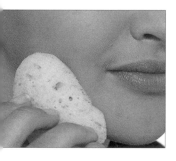

13 YELLOW TEETH

Visit your dentist or dental hygienist for regular check-ups and thorough cleaning to ensure your teeth are as white as possible, and bear in mind that yellow teeth tend to be stronger than whiter ones. To make them look whiter, avoid coral or brown-based lipsticks as the warm colours will emphasize the yellow tones in your teeth. Clear pink or red shades will make them appear whiter.

14 BLOODSHOT EYES

Red eyes are caused by the swelling of tiny blood vessels on the eye surface, from lack of sleep, excessive time spent in front of a computer or in a smoky atmosphere, or caused by an infection. If it's an ongoing problem, consult your doctor, or visit an optician for an eyesight examination to ensure there's no underlying cause.

For a quick temporary fix, use eye drops to bring the sparkle back to your eyes. These contain ingredients that will reduce the swelling in the blood vessels, decrease redness and cut down on dryness and itching.

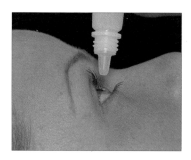

15 TIDEMARKS OF FOUNDATION

If you can see edges to the foundation on your chin, jawline or hairline, blend and soften them away with a damp cosmetic sponge. Do this in natural daylight so you can check the finished effect. Powder as usual afterwards.

16 UNHEALTHY NAILS

However strong nails are, their overall effect can be spoilt by clear or yellowing tips. A quick way to improve them is to run a white manicure pencil under the edges of the nails to give them a cleaner appearance. Combine with a coat of clear polish.

17 DROOPY EYES

To help lift droopy eyes, sweep a light-toned eyeshadow all over your eyelid. Apply a little eyeshadow with a clean cotton bud under your eyes, sweeping it slightly upwards. Apply extra coats of mascara on the lashes just above the iris of the eye to draw attention to the centre of your eye.

18 STRAGGLY EYEBROWS

Women often don't take much notice of their eyebrows until they look messy! The best plan is to tidy them with regular tweezing sessions. The ideal time is after a bath when your skin is warm and soft, the pores will be open from the heat and the hairs are easier to remove. Before bedtime is also good, so you don't have to face the day with blotchy skin.

First of all, use an eyebrow brush to sweep your brows into place, so that you can see their natural shape. Then pluck one hair at a time, always pulling in the direction of growth. First remove the hairs between your brows, and then thin out overall – generally, don't pluck above the eyebrow or you'll risk distorting the shape of your brows. The only exception is if there are hairs growing well above the natural browline. Finally, tweeze any stray hairs at the outer sides.

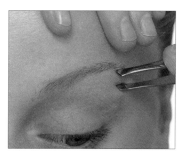

19 OVER-APPLIED BLUSHER

If you've forgotten to build up your blusher gradually, you may need to tone down an over-enthusiastic application of colour. The quickest and easiest way is to dust a little loose powder over the top of the problem area, until you've reached a softer blusher shade.

20 SORE EARS FROM EARRINGS

Try coating the posts of cheap earrings with hypo-allergenic clear nail polish. This should make them less likely to react with your sensitive skin. If your ears are sore, always give the skin plenty of time to heal up before wearing troublesome earrings again, and consider more expensive ones!

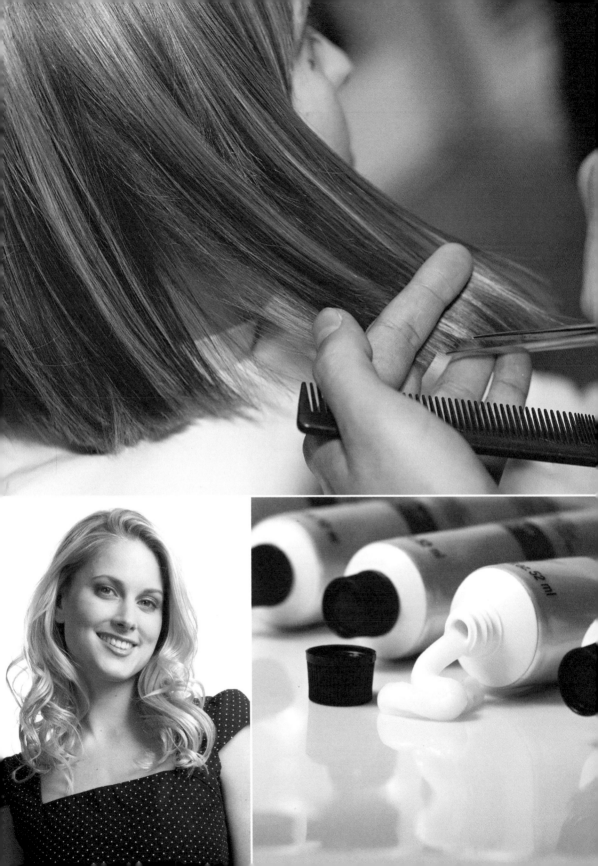

CARING FOR YOUR HAIR

Strong, shining hair is a valuable asset.
A daily haircare routine and prompt
treatment of any problems is vital to
boost and maintain the beauty of
healthy hair, while a good cut and
colour can transform the way you look
and feel about yourself.

SHAMPOOING HAIR

Establishing an efficient and effective haircare routine starts with great cleansing. Depending on whether you are washing daily or several times a week, and on the type and needs of your hair, there are several guides you can follow.

WHY SHAMPOO?

Designed to cleanse the hair and scalp, shampoos remove dirt without stripping away too much of the natural sebum, which provides shine. They generally contain cleansing agents, perfume, preservatives and conditioning agents that can coat the hair shaft to make it appear thicker. The conditioning agents smooth the cuticle scales to help prevent the hair from tangling and eliminate static electricity from the hair when it dries.

DIFFERENT TYPES OF SHAMPOO

There is a huge range of shampoos (some of which are called cleansers or hairbaths), so it's possible to find one suited to every hair type, texture, colour or condition. It is important that you change your shampoo according to different circumstances. For example, in the summer, use a moisturizing shampoo with a sun protection factor; when colouring, use a product to help prevent colour fade; or when suffering from a condition such as dandruff, opt for a specialist type.

THE PH FACTOR

This term refers to the acid/alkaline level of a substance. It is calculated on a scale of 1 to 14. Numbers below 7 denote acidity, while those over 7 indicate alkalinity.

Hair sebum has a pH factor of between 4.5 and 5.5, which is mildly acidic. Bacteria cannot survive in this pH, so it is important to maintain this protective layer of sebum in order to keep the skin, scalp and hair in optimum condition. If too acidic or too alkaline a product is used on hair, it may cause hair to become porous, weakened and even break.

Most shampoos range between a pH factor of 5 and 7; medicated varieties have a pH of about 7.3, which is near neutral.

Many shampoos are labelled 'pH balanced', and restore hair to its natural acidity, which is especially useful after chemical treatments such as colouring.

SCALP MASSAGE

Massage helps maintain a healthy scalp. It brings extra blood to the skin tissue, which enhances the delivery of nutrients and oxygen to the hair follicl Massage also reduces scalp tension – which can contribute to hair loss – loosens dead skin cells, and perhaps helps redress the overproduction of sebum, which makes hair oily.

You can easily give yourself a scalp massage at home. Use warm olive oil if the scalp is dry or tight. Try equal parts of witch hazel and mineral wate if you have an oily scalp. For a normal scalp, use equal parts rose and minera waters. Simply warm the chosen ointment in your hands, apply to the scalp evenly, then begin massaging your scalp at the hairline and work backwards to the base of your skull. Once you have reached the back, star again at your temples and work backwards. Use small, circular motions and medium pressure.

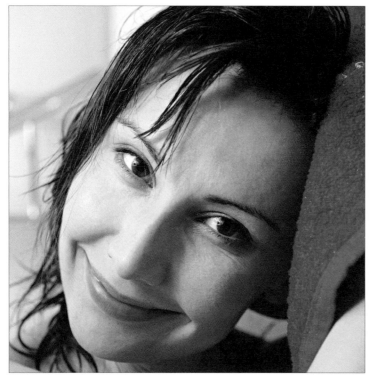

Left Hair looks and feels at its best when it clean, so try to make sure you wash it at lea every other day.

IPS FOR SHAMPOOING

Use the correct shampoo (and not too much) for your hair type. If in doubt, use the mildest shampoo you can buy.

Read the instructions for use first as every product varies slightly.

Buy sachets of shampoo to test which brand is the most suitable for your hair.

Don't wash your hair in the bath; dirty bath water is not conducive to clean hair. If you do choose to wash your hair in the tub, make sure you use the shower to rinse it through at the end.

Always wash your hairbrush and comb when you shampoo your hair.

Don't throw away a shampoo that doesn't lather. The amount of suds is determined by the active level of detergent and some shampoos create less suds than others, but this has no effect on their cleansing ability.

ERBAL SHAMPOO

Crush a few dried bay leaves with a rolling pin and mix with a handful of dried camomile flowers and a handful of rosemary. Place in a large jug and pour over 1 litre/1¾ pints/4 cups boiling water. Strain after 2–3 minutes and mix in 5ml/1 tsp of soft or liquid soap. Apply to the hair, massaging well for a minute or two. Rinse thoroughly.

INSES (AFTER SHAMPOOING)

Lemon juice added to the rinsing water will brighten blonde hair, while 30ml/ tbsp of cider vinegar added to rinsing water will add gloss and body to all hair.

Other rinses can be made up to treat a variety of problems. First you must make an infusion by placing 30ml/2 tbsp of a fresh herb in a china or glass bowl. Fresh herbs are best, but if you are using dried ones, remember they are stronger so you will need to halve the amount required for fresh herbs. Add 500ml/1 pint boiling water, cover and leave to steep for three hours. Strain before using. Try:

Southernwood to combat oiliness.
Nettle to stimulate hair growth.
Rosemary to prevent static.
Lavender to soothe a tight scalp.
Tea tree to ward off infestation.

shampooing hair

Taking care of healthy hair starts with a great cleansing routine. It's not rocket science but there is a technique to follow that means you will maintain maximum condition for your scalp and hair.

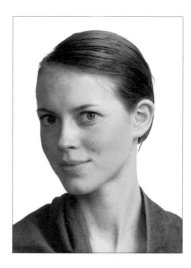

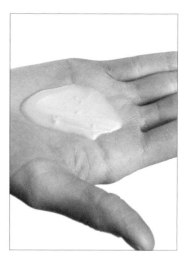

1 Wet hair thoroughly using a shower, ensuring all the layers are completely soaked through – this will activate the shampoo properly when it is applied.

2 Pour the shampoo into the palm of your hand, never directly on to the hair as it's tricky to control how much you use. For short hair you only need the same amount as a small coin, for longer hair you may require more, but never more than you can easily hold in the palm of your hand.

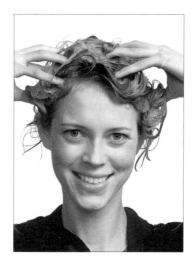

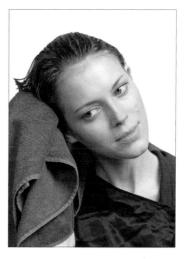

3 Work the shampoo through the hair, massaging your scalp and paying particular attention to the hairline around the ears and base of the neck. It should lather well but not too much.

4 Rinse away all the shampoo, then pat hair dry or squeeze gently to get rid of excess water. Don't rub or you will cause hair to tangle or break. Wet hair is more vulnerable than dry hair.

CONDITIONING HAIR

Hair in good condition is manageable, shiny, flexible and feels soft. Ideally, a simple shampoo would guarantee gorgeous results, but conditioning is often required to combat stresses caused by chemical processes, as well as to rectify problems.

WHY CONDITION

Glossy hair has cuticle scales that lie flat and overlap, reflecting light. Perming and colouring, rough handling and heat-styling all conspire to lift the cuticles and roughen them up, both allowing moisture to be lost from the cortex and making hair dry, lacklustre, and prone to tangle. Severely damaged cuticles break off completely, leaving the hair's cortex exposed, which leads to splits and breakages.

To put the shine back into hair and restore its natural lustre it may be necessary to use a specific conditioner that meets your hair's requirements. Conditioners, with the exception of hot oils, should be applied to freshly shampooed hair that has been blotted dry with a towel so that it is damp rather than wet.

DIFFERENT TYPES OF CONDITIONERS

Conditioning products are delivered in various different formats and have different effects:

• **Basic conditioners** coat the hair with a fine film, temporarily smoothing down the cuticle and making hair glossier and easier to manage. Leave on the hair for a few minutes before rinsing thoroughly.

• **Leave-in conditioners**, in spray or cream format, are intended to be applied after cleansing hair. Follow the instructions on the bottle carefully, then leave on the hair when drying and styling. They save time and are perfect for limited use when hair is extra-dry, after colouring, or when intense heat is used, but should not be used on a daily basis.

• **Conditioning sprays** are designed to be used prior to styling and form a protective barrier against the harmful effects of heat. They are also useful for reducing the amount of static electricity on flyaway hair.

• **Hot oils** give an intensive, deep nourishing treatment. To use, place the unopened tube in a cup of hot tap water and leave to heat for one minute. Next, wet the hair and towel it dry before twisting off the tube top. Massage the hot oil evenly into the scalp and throughout the hair for 1–3 minutes. For a more intensive treatment, cover the head with a shower cap and leave to penetrate. To finish, rinse the hair, then shampoo.

• **Intensive conditioning treatments** can be applied both in a salon – often as part of a ritual or service – or for occasional use at home. They may be rich crèmes or masques, and using them will help hair to retain its natural moisture balance, replenishing it where necessary. Use particularly if the hair is split, dry, frizzy, or difficult to manage.

• **Restructurants** penetrate the cortex, helping to repair and strengthen the inner part of damaged hair. They are helpful if hair is lank and limp and has lost its natural elasticity as a result of chemical treatments or physical damage.

• **Split-end treatments and serums** condition damaged hair. The best course of action for split ends is to have the ends trimmed, but this does not always solve the whole problem because the hair tends to break off and split at different levels. As an intermediate solution, split ends can appear to be temporarily sealed using these products.

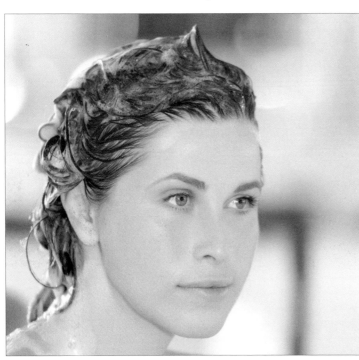

Left Heavier masques and crème treatments can be used on a once-a-week basis to restore hair's condition.

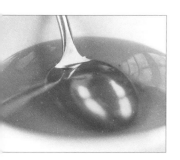

Above Natural ingredients such as honey and olive oil make nourishing hair masks.

Colour/perm conditioners are designed for chemically-treated hair. After-colour products add a protective film around porous areas of the hair, preventing colour loss. After-perm products help stabilize the hair, thus keeping the bounce in the curl.

NATURAL TREATMENTS FOR CONDITION AND SHINE:
Egg mask Blend two eggs with 30ml/ 2 tbsp water and 15ml/1 tbsp cider vinegar or lemon juice. Massage into damp hair and leave for 10–15 minutes before rinsing thoroughly with lukewarm (not hot) water.
Banana mask Mix together 1 mashed banana, 45ml/3 tbsp honey, 45ml/3 tbsp milk, 75ml/5 tbsp olive oil and 1 egg. Apply to damp hair and massage so it is evenly distributed. Leave on the hair for up to 30 minutes, then rinse thoroughly and shampoo and condition your hair as usual.
Yogurt mask Prepare by blending 105ml/7 tbsp plain (natural) yogurt with the beaten white of 1 egg. Apply to damp hair, massage through the roots to ends and leave for up to 30 minutes. Shampoo and condition your hair as usual.
Avocado, honey and olive oil are also great hair conditioners. You can use them in different combinations (use them in different combinations olive oil whisked with egg, or honey and olive oil blended in equal parts) or all together. Simply conjure up a consistency to suit you, leave on as long as you like to work their magic, and then shampoo and rinse hair well.

conditioning hair

Most hair that has been treated with a chemical process or exposed to environmental stresses will need either regular or occasional conditioning treatments after shampooing. Be careful not to apply too much conditioner – a little is designed to go a long way, and using too much product will make the hair feel lank and weighed down.

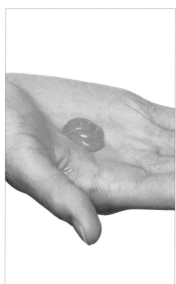

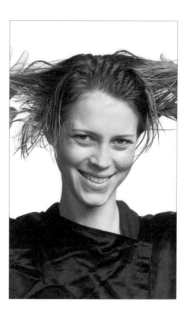

1 Follow the instructions on the packet, but as a general guide, use only a large coin-sized amount of product on mid-length hair, and less on shorter hair.

2 Rub the product lightly over the palms of both hands to make it easier to apply, then distribute it evenly along the lengths of damp (not soaking wet), cleansed hair.

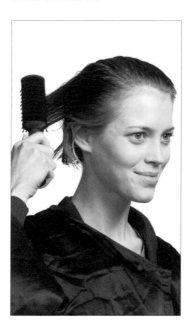

3 Work the product through the mid-lengths and ends rather than trying to massage it into the scalp, which is not usually necessary since the root area is new growth, which should be in a good condition naturally. Comb through hair gently using a wide-tooth comb to ensure the conditioner is evenly distributed. This type of comb is less likely to pull and break hair than other smaller-toothed combs. The conditioner should make it easy to detangle the hair. Wait the indicated amount of time (usually 2–5 minutes) to allow the conditioner to penetrate, before rinsing off with warm water. Towel dry, then comb again.

CHOOSING A STYLE

When it comes to choosing the perfect style, there are plenty of easy-to-follow guidelines on what cut best suits which face-shape, hair texture and type. But for all the advice, really the only rule is that you must feel confident and happy in yourself.

Fashions come and go with different trends and ideas, but essentially, if you learn to make the most of your looks by choosing a style that maximizes your best features, you will exude vitality and look beautiful because of it.

FACE SHAPES

Understanding your face shape will help get you started along the path to fabulous flattering hair. Is your face round, oval, square, heart-shaped or long? By defining your face shape and working with your stylist on a cut and style, you can minimize or emphasize different aspects of a face. Effects could include opening up the face and

making the best of small eyes, revealing a great eyebrow shape, softening a strong jaw-line or giving the illusion of shortening a long chin. A fringe (bangs) can also make you look younger and hide tell-tale wrinkles on the forehead.

If you are not sure what shape your face is, then the easiest way to find out is to draw the hair back off your face. Stand squarely in front of a mirror and use a lipstick to trace the outline of your face on to the mirror. When you stand back you should be able to see into which of the following categories your face shape falls: square, round, oval, heart-shaped or oblong.

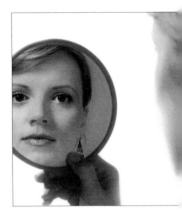

Above Take time to consider your face shape and which features you want to emphasize.

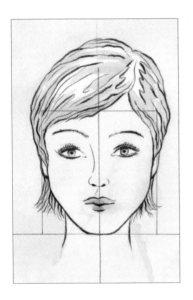

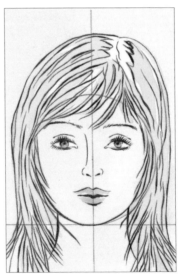

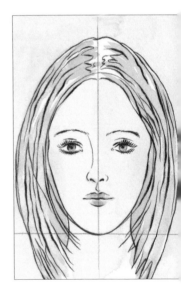

The square face is angular with a broad forehead and a square jawline. To make the best of this shape, choose a hairstyle with long layers, preferably one with gentle waves or curls, as these create a softness that detracts from the hard lines. Consider off-centre partings, loose curls and graduated cuts. Avoid blunt fringes (bangs).

On the round face, the distance between the forehead and the chin is about equal to the distance between the cheeks. Look at feathered haircuts where the hair falls forwards to slim down a fuller face. A short fringe (bangs) will seem to lengthen the face, while a shorter cut can be more flattering than a long style.

The oval face has wide cheekbones that taper down into a small, often pointed, chin, and up to a fairly narrow forehead. This is regarded by many experts as the perfect face shape, which looks good with almost any style. Now consider your facial features – do you prefer to emphasize your mouth, eyes, cheekbones or nose?

HE COMPLETE YOU

When choosing a new style you should also take into account your overall body shape and your personal lifestyle. If you are a traditional pear-shape, perhaps don't go for neat, elfin styles as they accentuate a small head and allow attention to be drawn to the lower half of your body, making your hips look even wider. Petite women might avoid styles with masses of very curly hair as this makes the head appear larger and out of proportion with the body.

If you wear glasses, choose frames and a hairstyle that complement each other. Large spectacles could spoil the look of a neat, feathery cut, while very fine frames could be overpowered by a voluminous style. Take your glasses to the salon when having your hair restyled, so that your stylist can take their shape into consideration.

To minimize signs of ageing, opt for a neater, more sophisticated cut, which can knock years off your look – leaving more tousled, casual styles to younger women. Don't get stuck in a style rut. Nothing is more dating than a tired look. Re-energize yourself with a new style from time to time. It doesn't have to be drastic, but a variation on a cut or colour works wonders.

FEATURE NOTES

You can use hairstyles to help disguise features that you don't particularly like:
• Prominent nose? Incorporate softness into your style.
• Pointed chin? Style the hair with width at the jawline.
• Low forehead? Choose a style with a wispy fringe, rather than one with a more full fringe.
• High forehead? Disguise a large forehead with a full fringe.
• Receding chin? Select a style that comes just below chin level, with waves or curls.
• Uneven hairline? A fringe should help conceal this problem.

THINKING AHEAD

It's important to plan where this new hairstyle will take you. If you fancy having a short crop, then consider how long it will take to grow out and what styles you might prefer in the future. It could make sense to go for a short one-length bob that grows out quite quickly rather than a close-cut style that will take longer to move into something else.

What about colour? Adopting a new block colour will mean regrowth coming through more obviously – so consider if you have the budget to continue having roots touched up, or whether highlights are a more practical way for you to change colour.

If you want a new look that requires more hair length or volume than you currently have, then discuss with your hairdresser ways that you can work towards achieving that look in a few months time. If you hate your fringe, then growing it out can take up to 12 months, but it's possible to have cuts and styles in the meantime that won't compromise your end goal.

When looking for a new style remember to consider:
• Why are you doing it? Is this really something you want to commit to?
• Do you have the right texture, volume and length of hair to achieve your desired style? In-salon consultations are free and talking with a hairdresser will give you a perspective on what is possible and what could suit you best.
• Are you going to need a new wardrobe to complement a new colour or cut?
• How much styling time will your new look require and are you prepared to invest that time?
• Get inspiration from looking at others around you, friends, magazines and celebrities. Remember, however, to think about how that style will look on you; don't be dazzled solely by how it looks on them.
• Where will this new style take you? If you've spent the past couple of years trying to grow out a fringe, then will this new style put you right back where you started, or is it halfway to the next look?

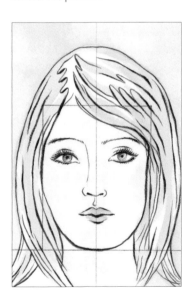

The heart-shaped face, where the widest point is at eye-level and then it tapers down to a neater chin shape, can be balanced by creating volume or width at chin level. A bob that flicks out just below the ears for example, can look fabulous. Or create volume at chin level with curls, layers or shattered perimeters.

The oblong face is characterized by a high forehead and long chin, and needs a haircut that gives the illusion of width to balance it. Soften the effect with short layers, or go for a bob with a fringe (bangs), which will create horizontal lines. Scrunch-dried or curly bobs balance a long face, too.

CUTTING HAIR

Being able to cut hair properly is a skill that requires great expertise. To create a desired shape, it's important to know where weight and bulk needs to be removed to achieve a good line and balance, emphasize good points and detract from bad ones.

Hair growth varies over different parts of the head, which means that your cut can appear out of shape quickly. As a general rule, a short, precision cut needs trimming every four weeks; a longer style every six to eight weeks. If you want to grow your hair long, it is essential to have it trimmed regularly – every three months – to keep the ends even. There are different ways to cut hair and it's a good idea to have some understanding of these in order to communicate with your hairdresser.

CLASSIC CUTS
Hairdressers learn the fundamental classic cuts, all of which can have variations to achieve different results:

• **The one-length bob** is also known as a pageboy. It's a haircut where the hair falls to a one-length point that is the same all the way round the head and usually sits above the shoulders.

Variations on a classic bob cut can then be used to individualize the look, such as making the front lengths longer than the back or vice versa. The hair is cut to form a smooth edge so that the lengths gradually rise or fall. It can be cut with or without a fringe (bangs) and with a central or side-parting. Hair can be blow-dried to curl out or under, or combed to hang straight.

• **A long one-length cut** is where hair falls to a point below the shoulders. Again it can be personalized with or

without a fringe and be blow-dried square-shaped or more rounded.

• **Layers** are where horizontal sections of hair are cut to the same length all round the head, so in effect the haircut mirrors the head shape with top layers falling to a higher point than lower layers. It is useful for thinning out thick hair and removing bulk. You can have layers any length, from short to long.

• **Graduation** is a technique used to create top layers which are shorter than underneath layers. You can create a greater or lesser degree of graduation or create reverse graduation where underneath layers are shorter than top layers. It's an important technique for shaping styles.

• **A square-layered cut** is sometimes called box layers or graduated layers, and combines layering and graduation. It's called a square layer because if all the hair were blown back off the face it would form a square shape.

• **A round layered cut**, also called a French crop, is a basic layered shape where the hair is cut into rounded layers, creating a softer end shape.

CUTTING TECHNIQUES
Ways of cutting hair vary according to the effect you want to achieve, but there are several basic techniques that a hairdresser is likely to use:

• **Blunt cutting** is when the ends of the hair are cut straight across and is often used for hair of one length or definite lines.

• **Point cutting** is where the scissors are pointed into the haircut to break up straight lines and add texture.

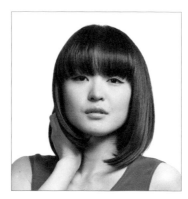
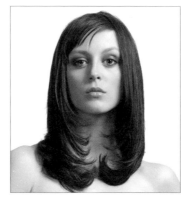
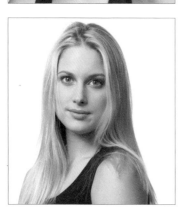

Clockwise, from top left Graduated cut with a fringe (bangs); long bob with a fringe; layered hair with a short fringe; long one-length hair.

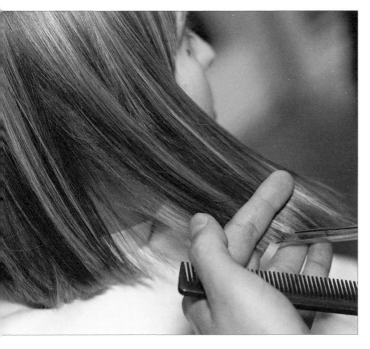

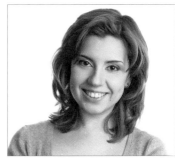

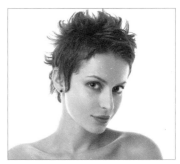

Above Angling scissors will cut either blunt lines or chip into the ends of the hair, creating different finished effects.

• **Slide cutting** is a way to thin thick hair and give a soft finish. This technique is often done when the hair is dry using open scissors to slice the hair.
• **Razor cutting** is literally using a razor rather than scissors, and creates softness, tapering, and internal movement so that the hair moves freely. It can also be used instead of scissors to shorten hair.
• **Thinning** is done either with thinning scissors or a razor; it removes bulk and weight without affecting the overall length of the hair and is ideal for very heavy, thick hair.

CLEVER CUTS

The art of hairdressing is in applying different techniques and cuts to make the most of a client's hair type and texture and achieve a look that suits their appearance and lifestyle. These are some of the most common tricks of the trade:
• Fine, thin, flyaway hair can be given volume and movement by blunt cutting.
• Mid-length hair can benefit tremendously from being lightly layered to give extra volume.
• Short, thin hair can be blunt cut and the edges graduated to give movement.
• Some hairdressers razor-cut fine hair to give a thicker and more voluminous effect. It is best not to let fine hair grow too long. As soon as it reaches the shoulders it tends to look wispy.
• Thick and coarse hair can be controlled by reducing the weight to give more style. Avoid very short styles because the hair will stick out. Try a layered cut with movement.
• Layering also helps achieve height and eliminates weight. On shorter styles, the weight can be reduced with thinning scissors expertly used on the ends only.

Top A widow's peak can look very attractive if the hair is cut in a style that suits the shape of the face.
Above Cowlicks can be difficult to style or tame, so it is important that the hairdresser thinks carefully about how to cut the hair.

STYLING PROBLEMS

Sometimes hair grows in different directions, which may cause various styling problems.
• A **cowlick** is found on the front hairline and occurs when the hair grows in a swirl, backwards and then forwards. Clever cutting can redistribute the weight and go some way to solving this problem.
• A **double crown** occurs when there are two pivots of natural hair at the top of the head, rather than the usual one, causing hair to grow forwards, making it difficult to tie back. Styles with height at the crown or that incorporate a fringe are most suitable.
• A **widow's peak** is a descending point on the hairline, forming a V-shape, usually above the forehead. Taking hair in the reverse direction to the growth will give the impression of a natural wave that will frame a face.

COLOURING HAIR

Beautiful hair is about condition and colour. You may be blessed with fantastic natural colour but still fancy a change, or maybe your own colouring needs a boost. Perhaps you like to change your hair tone as often as your clothes. The good news is, you can!

Technological advances in the past few years mean that hair colorants have never been better, both in terms of product efficiency and colour choice. You can now choose between temporary, semi-permanent, demi-permanent and permanent colour, each offers a different lasting power depending on the base or natural colour, of your hair.

DIFFERENT SHADES

Professional hair colours are made up of codes which follow an international numbering system. The first number refers to your natural hair colour, or base, and is counted from 0 (a natural blue/black) to 9 (extra light blonde). After a point, a second number indicates the tone of the hair. For instance, .0 is matt while .7 is violet. A third number indicates a secondary tone. So 6 will be Dark Blonde, while 6.4 indicates Dark Copper Blonde and 6.46 denotes Dark Copper Red Blonde.

It's not necessary to learn the numbering system but it can be useful to ask your hairdresser which numbers they have applied to create the colour you prefer.

SKIN TEST

It's vital to do a skin test before using any colorant as some people are allergic to ingredients such as para-dyes, which appear in many products. An allergic reaction can range from mild itching to severe burning. Hairdressers should insist on doing a skin test 24 hours before applying colorants (beware any salons that don't) and most good products for home use now include a skin test, which you must perform. A small amount of product should be applied to a clean pulse point – behind the ear or in the crook of the elbow – and left for a minimum of 24 hours to check for any bad or allergic reaction.

PERMANENT COLOURS

These colorants, or tints as they are often called, lighten or darken, and can very effectively cover white. While the colour is permanent, don't forget that roots will need retouching every 4–6 weeks to keep pace with new growth.

Permanent colorant works by putting colour pigment mixed with hydrogen peroxide into the cortex (the centre) of the hair shaft during the development time. The pigment adds melanin for darker shades of brown and black, and pheomelanin for red and yellow shades. After the colorant is applied, the oxygen in the developer swells the pigments in the colorant until they comprise such large molecules that they can't escape from the cortex and so are locked in.

Another way of permanently changing hair colour is by lightening it using bleach with hydrogen peroxide

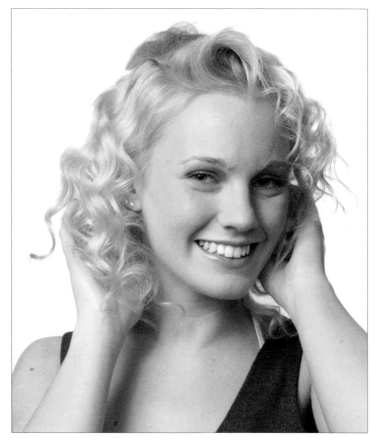

Left The colouring process can enhance the natural shine and condition of your hair, leaving it healthy and attractive-looking.

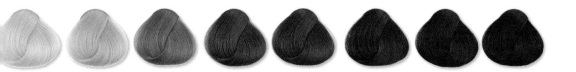

o activate the bleach) to de-colour
he hair, creating a very light blonde. The
eroxide enters the hair shaft by means
f ammonia which lifts the cuticles.
nce inside, the peroxide zaps the
olour pigment in the hair, making it as
ght as you want. It's a harsh treatment
o gentle aftercare is essential. Over-
leaching will destroy the hair so be
areful. For this reason, it's wise to get
professional to do a lightening process.

EMI-PERMANENT COLOURS
hese are more gentle than permanent
olorants as there is no ammonia or
ydrogen peroxide to help the pigment
enetrate the cortex. Instead, while it is
bsorbed into the cuticle layer and into
he cortex, it stays only until it is
vashed out. The effect can only be
sed to add, enrich, or darken hair
olour (semi-permanents cannot make
air any lighter). The colour fades
radually, washing away over several
hampoos (12–20 depending on the

elow Hair colour is applied via different
echniques. Foils are a great way of putting
ne highlights through hair.

manufacturer and the type of hair).
They are ideal for those who don't
want to commit to a permanent
change; for blending in grey hairs;
and for conditioning hair.

DEMI-PERMANENT COLOURS
Halfway between a permanent and a
semi-permanent, demi-permanent
colorant includes a small amount of
hydrogen peroxide but no ammonia.
It won't change the existing pigment
but it will deposit more colour in the
hair shaft, enhancing natural colour
and covering grey. There isn't such
obvious regrowth as with permanent
treatments, since colour is added rather
then altered, and it's kinder than
permanent colour. However, it will still
only last up to 20 washes.

TEMPORARY COLOURS
These are mild colorants that last
about 1–5 washes, depending on the
porosity of the hair. They work by

Below Colorants can be mixed to create
virtually any shade, tone and intensity you
desire. Professional colourists are true artists.

Above There is a wide range of natural tones
to choose from when you are looking for a
new colour, as this colour swatch demonstrates.

coating the outside, or cuticle layer,
of the hair but do not penetrate the
cortex as there is no hydrogen peroxide
in them. However, if the hair is
damaged and the cuticle open, parts
of the hair can trap colour molecules.
In this case, hair must be conditioned
and the cuticle smoothed before
applying. Temporary colours are good
for a quick change or for counteracting
discoloration. They come in mousse,
hairspray, setting lotion, gel, glitter
dust or cream formulations.

DID YOU KNOW?
• Colouring swells the hair shaft,
making fine hair appear thicker.
• Colour changes the porosity of the
hair and can help combat greasiness.
• Rich tones reflect more light and
give hair a thicker appearance.
• Highlights give fine hair extra
texture and break up thick hair.

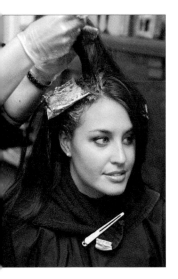

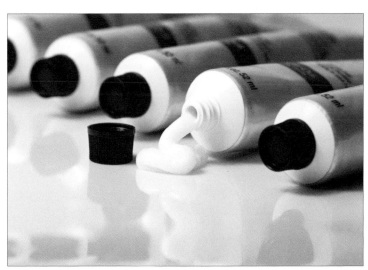

INDEX

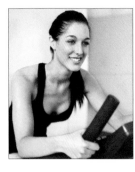

Picture Credits
iStock: 1, 2, 6t, 7t, 8b, 10br,
11bl, 11bcl, 12, 13, 14, 15bl,
15bcl, 15bcr, 22t, 24b, 68br, 70l,
71r, 73, 81tr, 84br, 85br, 87c,
87r, 88br, 89br, 90tl, 91br, 92tl,
93tl, 97tl, 98tl, 100tl, 102tl,
103tl, 105tl, 109tl, 110t, 135tl,
141tl, 141c, 144t, 144br, 146b,
148b, 150t, 153, 155, 158

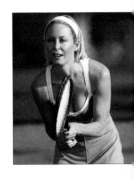